T0131009

Causes of Sleep Complaints

Editors

KEITH ROMEO A. AGUILERA

AGNES T. REMULLA

SLEEP MEDICINE CLINICS

www.sleep.theclinics.com

March 2022 • Volume 17 • Number 1

ELSEVIER

1600 John F. Kennedy Boulevard • Suite 1800 • Philadelphia, Pennsylvania, 19103-2899

http://www.theclinics.com

SLEEP MEDICINE CLINICS Volume 17, Number 1
March 2022, ISSN 1556-407X, ISBN-13: 978-0-323-84981-4

Editor: Joanna Collett
Developmental Editor: Axell Ivan Jade M. Purificacion

© **2022 Elsevier Inc. All rights reserved.**

This periodical and the individual contributions contained in it are protected under copyright by Elsevier, and the following terms and conditions apply to their use:

Photocopying
Single photocopies of single articles may be made for personal use as allowed by national copyright laws. Permission of the Publisher and payment of a fee is required for all other photocopying, including multiple or systematic copying, copying for advertising or promotional purposes, resale, and all forms of document delivery. Special rates are available for educational institutions that wish to make photocopies for non-profit educational classroom use. For information on how to seek permission visit www.elsevier.com/permissions or call: (+44) 1865 843830 (UK)/(+1) 215 239 3804 (USA).

Derivative Works
Subscribers may reproduce tables of contents or prepare lists of articles including abstracts for internal circulation within their institutions. Permission of the Publisher is required for resale or distribution outside the institution. Permission of the Publisher is required for all other derivative works, including compilations and translations (please consult www.elsevier.com/permissions).

Electronic Storage or Usage
Permission of the Publisher is required to store or use electronically any material contained in this periodical, including any article or part of an article (please consult www.elsevier.com/permissions). Except as outlined above, no part of this publication may be reproduced, stored in a retrieval system or transmitted in any form or by any means, electronic, mechanical, photocopying, recording or otherwise, without prior written permission of the Publisher.

Notice
No responsibility is assumed by the Publisher for any injury and/or damage to persons or property as a matter of products liability, negligence or otherwise, or from any use or operation of any methods, products, instructions or ideas contained in the material herein. Because of rapid advances in the medical sciences, in particular, independent verification of diagnoses and drug dosages should be made. Although all advertising material is expected to conform to ethical (medical) standards, inclusion in this publication does not constitute a guarantee or endorsement of the quality or value of such product or of the claims made of it by its manufacturer.

Sleep Medicine Clinics (ISSN 1556-407X) is published quarterly by Elsevier Inc., 360 Park Avenue South, New York, NY 10010-1710. Months of issue are March, June, September and December. Business and Editorial Offices: 1600 John F. Kennedy Blvd., Ste. 1800, Philadelphia, PA 19103-2899. Customer Service Office: 3251 Riverport Lane, Maryland Heights, MO 63043. Periodicals postage paid at New York, NY and additional mailing offices. Subscription prices are $234.00 per year (US individuals), $100.00 (US and Canadian students), $653.00 (US institutions), $272.00 (Canadian individuals), $267.00 (international individuals) $135.00 (International students), $682.00 (Canadian and International institutions). Foreign air speed delivery is included in all *Clinics* subscription prices. All prices are subject to change without notice. **POSTMASTER:** Send change of address to *Sleep Medicine Clinics*, Elsevier Health Sciences Division, Subscription Customer Service, 3251 Riverport Lane, Maryland Heights, MO 63043. Customer Service: **Tel: 1-800-654-2452 (U.S. and Canada); 314-447-8871 (outside U.S. and Canada). Fax: 314-447-8029. E-mail: journalscustomerservice-usa@elsevier.com (for print support); journalsonline-support-usa@elsevier.com (for online support).**

Reprints. For copies of 100 or more of articles in this publication, please contact the Commercial Reprints Department, Elsevier Inc., 360 Park Avenue South, New York, NY 10010-1710. Tel.: 212-633-3874; Fax: 212-633-3820; E-mail: reprints@elsevier.com.

Sleep Medicine Clinics is covered in *MEDLINE/PubMed (Index Medicus)*.

SLEEP MEDICINE CLINICS

SERIES OF RELATED INTEREST

Neurologic Clinics
Available at: https://www.neurologic.theclinics.com/

THE CLINICS ARE AVAILABLE ONLINE!
Access your subscription at:
www.theclinics.com

Contributors

CONSULTING EDITORS

TEOFILO LEE-CHIONG Jr, MD
Professor of Medicine, National Jewish Health,
Professor of Medicine, University of Colorado,
Denver, Colorado, USA; Chief Medical Liaison,
Philips Respironics, Pennsylvania, USA

ANA C. KRIEGER, MD
Chief, Division of Sleep Neurology Medical
Director, Weill Cornell Center for Sleep
Medicine, New York, Professor of Clinical
Medicine, Professor of Medicine in Neurology
and Genetic Medicine, New York, USA

EDITORS

KEITH ROMEO A. AGUILERA, MD
Center Head, Comprehensive Sleep Disorders
Center, Assistant Training Officer, Department
of Otolaryngology–Head and Neck Surgery, St.
Luke's Medical Center, Global City,
Philippines; Program Director, Sleep Medicine
Fellowship Program, St. Luke's Medical
Center, Global City and Quezon City,
Philippines; Assistant Professor 1, St. Luke's
Medical Center–College of Medicine, Quezon
City, Philippines

AGNES T. REMULLA, MD
Head, Sleep Laboratory, Asian Hospital and
Medical Center, Muntinlupa City, Philippines;
Director, Philippine Board of Otolaryngology–
Head and Neck Surgery, Associate Clinical
Professor, Assistant Chair for Teaching,
Department of Otolaryngology–Head and Neck
Surgery, University of the Philippines–
Philippine General Hospital, Manila, Philippines

AUTHORS

CHUN TING AU, PhD
Department of Paediatrics, Faculty of
Medicine, The Chinese University of Hong
Kong, Hong Kong SAR, China; Department of
Paediatrics, Princes of Wales Hospital, Shatin,
Hong Kong, China

**RYLENE A. BAQUILOD, MD, FPCP, FPCCP,
FPSSM**
Active Staff, Pulmonary and Pulmonary Critical
Care, Chong Hua Hospital, Cebu City,
Philippines

REINZI LUZ S. BAUTISTA, MD, FPSOHNS
Sleep Medicine Fellow, Ear Nose Throat –
Head and Neck Surgery (ENT-HNS) Specialist,
Comprehensive Sleep Disorders Center, St.
Luke's Medical Center – Global City, Taguig
City, Philippines

NGAN YIN CHAN, PhD
Li Chiu Kong Family Sleep Assessment Unit,
Department of Psychiatry, Faculty of Medicine,
The Chinese University of Hong Kong, Hong
Kong SAR, China; Department of Psychiatry,
Shatin Hospital, Ma On Shan, Hong Kong,
China

JAHYEON CHO, MD
Department of Psychiatry, Dream Sleep Clinic,
Seoul, South Korea

WEERASAK CHONCHAIYA, MD
Professor, Head of Maximizing Thai Children's
Developmental Potential Research Unit, Head
of Division of Growth and Development,
Department of Pediatrics, King Chulalongkorn
Memorial Hospital, Faculty of Medicine,
Chulalongkorn University, Pathumwan District,
Bangkok, Thailand

TRIPAT DEEP SINGH, MBBS, MD, RPSGT, RST, CCSH
Director of Academy of Sleep Wake Science India, Chief Medical Officer, REM42, International Sleep Specialist, World Sleep Federation Program

RAVI GUPTA, MD, PhD
Departments of Neurology and Psychiatry, Division of Sleep Medicine, All India Institute of Medical Sciences, Rishikesh, India

APRIL FATIMA J. HERNANDEZ, MD, DSBPP, FPSSM
Sleep Specialist – Psychiatrist, Comprehensive Sleep Disorders Center, St. Luke's Medical Center – Quezon City, Department of Psychiatry, University of the East Ramon Magsaysay Memorial Medical Center, Quezon City, Philippines; Comprehensive Sleep Disorders Center, St. Luke's Medical Center – Global City, Taguig City, Philippines

NIRAJ KUMAR, MD, DM
Departments of Neurology and Psychiatry, Division of Sleep Medicine, All India Institute of Medical Sciences, Rishikesh, India

JI HYUN LEE, MD
Department of Psychiatry, Dream Sleep Clinic, Seoul, South Korea

SHIRLEY XIN LI, PhD, DClinPsy
Department of Psychology, The State Key Laboratory of Brain and Cognitive Sciences, The University of Hong Kong, Hong Kong SAR, China

SOMPRASONG LIAMSOMBUT, MD
Division of Pulmonary and Critical Care, Department of Medicine, Ramathibodi Hospital, Ramathibodi Hospital Sleep Disorder Center, Mahidol University, Bangkok, Thailand

ALBERT L. RAFANAN, MD, FCCP, FASSM, FPSSM, FPCP, FPCCP, DABSM
Assistant Medical Director for Continuing Medical Education, Unit Head, Center for Sleep Disorders, Chairman, Critical Care Committee, Chong Hua Hospital, Professor of Medicine, Cebu Doctors University College of Medicine, Cebu City, Philippines

CRISTINE CELINE TAN, MD, DPBOHNS
Sleep Medicine Fellow, Ear Nose Throat - Head and Neck Surgery (ENT-HNS) Specialist, Comprehensive Sleep Disorders Center, St. Luke's Medical Center – Quezon City, Quezon City, Philippines

VISASIRI TANTRAKUL, MD
Ramathibodi Hospital Sleep Disorder Center, Division of Sleep Medicine, Department of Medicine, Ramathibodi Hospital, Mahidol University, Bangkok, Thailand

RIMAWATI TEDJASUKMANA, MD, PhD, RPSGT
Lecturer, Department of Neurology, Universitas Kristen Krida Wacana (Krida Wacana Christian University), Head of Sleep and Snoring Clinic, Staff Neurologist, Medistra Hospital, Jakarta, Indonesia

MONTIDA VEERAVIGROM, MD
Assistant Professor, Section of Child Neurology, Department of Pediatrics, The University of Chicago, Biological Sciences, Chicago, Illinois, USA

YUN KWOK WING, FRCPsych
Li Chiu Kong Family Sleep Assessment Unit, Department of Psychiatry, Faculty of Medicine, The Chinese University of Hong Kong, Hong Kong SAR, China; Department of Psychiatry, Shatin Hospital, Ma On Shan, Hong Kong, China

YOKE-YEOW YAP, MD, MMed (ORL-HNS)
KPJ Johor Specialist Hospital, Johor Bahru, Malaysia

Contents

Around 21% of workers reported working on shifts in 2017, and consequently, shift workers experience multiple sleep disturbances such as excessive sleepiness, insomnia, sleep deprivation, and social jet lag. These eventually lead to shift work disorder or exacerbation of other sleep disorders such as insomnia, obstructive sleep apnea, restless legs syndrome, and nonrapid eye movement parasomnia. Despite multiple interventions and guidelines, poor compliance to treatment is often encountered due to temporary relief of sleep disturbances provided by the treatment. Hence there is a need for comprehensive evaluation of those individuals who need to be awake during the night and asleep during the day.

Sleep is vital to life, even when women enter into pregnancy state. Good sleep is important for a healthy pregnancy. Sleep disturbances are common during pregnancy and can be due to the change of pregnancy itself or the results of sleep disorders. There is growing evidence linking sleep disturbances with adverse maternal and fetal outcomes. Differentiation of sleep disorders in order to provide appropriate treatment as well as promoting good sleep for pregnant women is important. A multidisciplinary team to provide sleep care during antenatal period may be needed.

Snoring can be harmless (primary) or a symptom of sleep-disordered breathing (secondary) and should alert the physician to evaluate the patient for risks thereof. Phenotypes of snoring and sleep-disordered breathing (SDB) are anatomic and nonanatomic and identifying these phenotypes and their interrelationships are critical to effective therapy. Mouth breathing alerts the physician to nasal airway obstruction, signals orofacial growth changes in children, and heralds the progression of SDB. Systematic evaluation to establish phenotypes includes assessing sleep habits, comorbidities, upper airway examination, polysomnography, and drug-induced sleep endoscopy. Strategies for treatment should be personalized and precise to the phenotype(s) to achieve the most benefit.

The COVID-19 pandemic affected sleep in several people. Though most of the studies argued that age, gender, employment, finances, responsibilities, and exposure to sunlight governed sleep-wake schedule and sleep disturbances, there is also scientific evidence to suggest that these issues could have aroused because of the infiltration of the central nervous system (CNS) by SARS-CoV-2. Sleep disturbances must be addressed during the pandemic as sleep disturbances and systemic inflammation run in a vicious cycle; quality of sleep and timing of vaccination can influence the immune response to vaccination and subjects having obstructive sleep apnea (OSA) are at higher risk for having SARS-CoV-2 infection-related complications.

Sleep complaints are common among children. These include both night-time and daytime symptoms, such as trouble falling asleep, problems in maintaining sleep, snoring, and unusual events during sleep and daytime functioning impairment. However, sleep complaints in children are often overlooked and undertreated in clinical practice. Untreated sleep problems may further impact on children's development and will persist into adulthood in some cases. This review summarizes the common sleep complaints and disorders in school children, and provides an overview of the epidemiology, clinical features, consequences, and treatment of the sleep problems.

Pediatric insomnia is relatively common in general pediatric practice and has an even higher prevalence in those with neurodevelopmental disorders. Detailed sleep history, sleep diary, associated daytime symptoms, and factors contributing to insomnia should be thoroughly evaluated to determine the diagnosis and further plan for management. Behavioral management should be the first step for the management of insomnia in children and adolescents. Although there is no FDA-approved medication for the treatment of insomnia in children, some medications may be prescribed with caution, particularly if behavioral management is not effective, in selected conditions, and if the benefits outweigh the risks.

Genetic factors are surmised to regulate sleep as evidenced by the heritability of sleep traits, specific genetic polymorphisms of these traits, and familial sleep disorders. Sleep is also a very complex behavior that is regulated by circadian rhythm, homeostatic drive, and other processes. All these processes appear to have genetic factors; however, we still cannot elucidate sleep genes. Recent studies in humans and animal models have uncovered some genetic factors underlying sleep disturbances. In this review, we present an overview of genetical regulation of sleep and genetic factors underlying several sleep disturbances.

Sleep-disordered breathing (SDB) is highly prevalent in patients with heart failure (HF). Untreated obstructive sleep apnea (OSA) and central sleep apnea (CSA) in patients with HF are associated with worse outcomes. Detailed sleep history along with polysomnography (PSG) should be conducted if SDB is suspected in patients with HF. First line of treatment is the optimization of medical therapy for HF and if symptoms persist despite optimization of the treatment, positive airway pressure (PAP) therapy will be started to treat SDB. At present, there is limited evidence to prescribe any drugs for treating CSA in patients with HF. There is limited evidence for the efficacy of continuous positive airway pressure (CPAP) or adaptive servo-ventilation (ASV) in improving mortality in patients with heart failure with reduced ejection fraction (HFrEF). There is a need to perform well-designed studies to identify different phenotypes of CSA/OSA in patients with HF and to determine which phenotype responds to which therapy. Results of ongoing trials, ADVENT-HF, and LOFT-HF are eagerly awaited to shed more light on the management of CSA in patients with HF. Until then the management of SDB in patients with HF is limited due to the lack of evidence and guidance for treating SDB in patients with HF.

This review presents the normal physiologic changes in ventilation during sleep and how they can be detrimental to chronic obstructive pulmonary disease (COPD). Sleep-related breathing disorders (SRBDs) in COPD lead to higher morbidity and mortality if left unrecognized and untreated. The diagnosis of SRBDs requires a high index of suspicion, as symptoms may overlap with other sleep disorders. Mortality risk is improved when patients with Obstructive Sleep Apnea (overlap syndrome) are treated with positive airway pressure and when long-term nocturnal noninvasive ventilation is started on chronic stable hypercapnic COPD. Treatment of isolated nocturnal oxygen desaturation has not been associated with improved survival.

Sleep and appetite have a circadian tendency with a diurnal rhythm. There is a reciprocal interaction between sleep and obesity. Having poor sleep, in either amount or timing, is associated with difficulty in controlling appetite, resulting in obesity. Being overweight or obese increases the risk of developing sleep disorders such as obstructive sleep apnea, which may further impair sleep quality. Sleep in children and adolescents plays an important role in cognitive, emotional, and physical development. Sleep problems in this age group are linked to obesity, which leads to metabolic syndrome, diabetes, or hypertension in the early stages of life.

Preface
Waking Up to Sleep

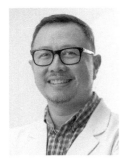
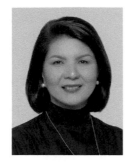

Keith Romeo A. Aguilera, MD   Agnes T. Remulla, MD

Editors

The field of sleep medicine is enjoying much attention in recent decades and more attention the past couple of years. A quick search of "sleep" in PubMed yields a steeply rising number of published studies, the highest of which was in 2021 at more than 23,000.[1] The relevance of sleep in basic and clinical research, particularly how this can transcend to our daily lives, makes looking into sleep much more pertinent. We now understand that a balance of events occurring while awake and asleep determines our general health and quality of life. Therefore, the timing of the peak number of published studies related to sleep reflects the current concerns regarding understanding sleep, its disorders, and how to manage the roughly 70 disorders listed in the third edition of the *International Classification of Sleep Disorders* (2014).[2]

The COVID-19 pandemic has isolated many and removed numerous zeitgebers that we had unknowingly relied upon. Prolonged lifestyle change and its effect on daily activities and sleep highlight the importance of understanding sleep disorders. Determining the cause of the most common sleep complaints is therefore essential. Children and adults alike experience sleep disorders. These may be related to physiologic, genetic, situational, or lifestyle determinants. Demands of school and work do not always agree with our sleep requirements. Stress, natural sleep propensity, preexisting sleep disorders, and medical comorbidities coupled with maladaptive responses may result in detrimental sleep effects.

With the increasing volume of available research, organized and curated information is valuable to every clinician. In this issue, esteemed sleep specialists of different medical fields review the most common causes of sleep disorders, approaches to evaluation, and its subsequent management.

Keith Romeo A. Aguilera, MD
Room 308, Medical Arts Building
St. Luke's Medical Center
32nd Street, Corner 5th Avenue
Bonifacio Global City, Taguig City
Philippines 1634

Agnes T. Remulla, MD
Unit 420, Medical Office Building
Asian Hospital and Medical Center
2205 Civic Drive
Alabang, Muntinlupa
Metro Manila, Philippines 1780

E-mail addresses:
kaaguilera@stlukes.com.ph (K.R.A. Aguilera)
antironaremulla@up.edu.ph (A.T. Remulla)

REFERENCES

1. Available at: https://pubmed.ncbi.nlm.nih.gov/?term=sleep&filter=years.2021-2021&sort=date&size=20. Accessed.
2. American Academy of Sleep Medicine. International classification of sleep disorders. 3rd ed. Darien (IL): American Academy of Sleep Medicine; 2014.

Sleep Med Clin 17 (2022) xi
https://doi.org/10.1016/j.jsmc.2021.12.001
1556-407X/22/© 2021 Published by Elsevier Inc.

Sleep Disturbances During Shift Work

April Fatima J. Hernandez, MD, DSBPP, FPSSM[a,b,c],*, Reinzi Luz S. Bautista, MD, FPSOHNS[b], Cristine Celine Tan, MD, DPBOHNS[a]

KEYWORDS

- Shift work • Sleep disturbances • Circadian desynchronization • Circadian rhythm • Insomnia
- Sleep deprivation • Social jet lag • Shift work disorder

KEY POINTS

- Shift work may lead to circadian misalignment, which is associated with numerous medical conditions and sleep disorders.
- Circadian misalignment has been found to be involved in the development of metabolic and cardiovascular health problems.
- Sleep disturbances, such as excessive sleepiness, insomnia, sleep deprivation, and social jet lag, are evident among shift workers and contribute to the development of sleep disorders.
- Most shift workers find it difficult to comply with behavioral interventions, as they provide only transient improvement in sleep.

INTRODUCTION

A substantial proportion of the working population is involved in shift work. In the 2017 update of the European Working Conditions Survey, 21% of all workers reported working in shifts, with most working in alternating or rotating shifts.[1] The US Department of Labor reported that during the period 2017 to 2018, 16% of wage and salary workers in the United States worked a nondaytime schedule, including 6% who worked evenings and 4% who worked nights.[2]

Shift work is regarded as any work schedule outside of the regular daytime hours.[3] As an employment strategy, shift work allows for the round-the-clock operation of many services and industries. Shift work schedules can vary enormously from industry to industry but are nonetheless regulated by existing labor laws.

Shifts can be identified by their typical start times: night shift workers have regular start times between 6 PM and 4 AM, early morning shift workers start between 4 AM and 7 AM, and evening/afternoon shift workers start between 2 PM and 6 PM (Fig. 1).[4] Early morning shift work is the most common alternate work shift. Rotating shift workers have a revolving schedule along the various start times. The rotation of shifts can be fast or slow (Fig. 2) and can occur in a clockwise or counterclockwise direction as opposed to permanent or fixed work schedules (Fig. 3).[5,6]

Because of the increasing number of individuals working on different types of shifts, research for the past 2 decades have focused on the effects of shift work on the individual's health (Fig. 4). They are potentially at increased risk for a variety of health problems due to the disturbance in their sleep,[7] which include metabolic syndrome and cardiovascular disease.[8] Gender could be an influence on this relationship, as female shift workers have been shown to have a higher risk of developing metabolic syndrome but surprisingly have

[a] Comprehensive Sleep Disorders Center, St. Luke's Medical Center – Quezon City, 279 E. Rodriguez Sr. Avenue, Quezon City 1112, Philippines; [b] Comprehensive Sleep Disorders Center, St. Luke's Medical Center – Global City, Rizal Drive cor. 32nd St. and 5th Avenue, Taguig City 1634, Philippines; [c] Department of Psychiatry, University of the East Ramon Magsaysay Memorial Medical Center, Aurora Boulevard, Quezon City 1105, Philippines
* Corresponding author. Comprehensive Sleep Disorders Center, St. Luke's Medical Center – Quezon City, 279 E. Rodriguez Sr. Avenue, Quezon City 1112, Philippines.
E-mail address: afjhernandez@stlukes.com.ph

Sleep Med Clin 17 (2022) 1–10
https://doi.org/10.1016/j.jsmc.2021.10.001
1556-407X/22/© 2021 Elsevier Inc. All rights reserved.

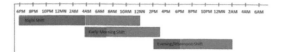

Fig. 1. Shift work schedules with corresponding typical start times are indicated by the blue bars. Normal 8 hours of work indicated by the orange bars. (*Data from* Drake and Wright[4].)

a lower risk of diabetes mellitus and hypertension compared with male shift workers. Rotating shift schedule was associated with an increased risk of diabetes and hypertension compared with other types of shift schedule; however, permanent night shift workers were shown to be at higher risk of

developing obesity than rotating shift workers. Shift work was also associated with an increased risk of coronary artery disease and ischemic heart disease. Self-reports[9] of acne vulgaris, seborrheic dermatitis and atopic dermatitis, skin dryness, and pruritic symptoms were more prevalent among Filipino call center agents who were described as poor sleepers. Working the night shift tends to disrupt secretion of hormones, increasing the risk for breast and prostate cancer, gastrointestinal abnormalities, and reproductive aberrations.[10]

Aside from the medical conditions observed among shift workers, sleep disturbances are common among this population. Around 50 to 70 million Americans suffer from sleep disorders that are associated with deleterious health

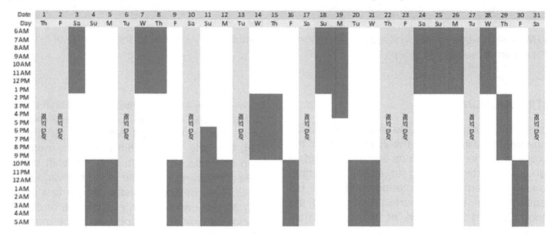

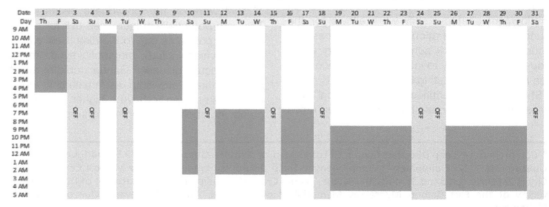

Fig. 2. Fast versus slow clockwise rotating shifts. (*A*) Sample 30-day schedule of a bedside nurse in a private tertiary hospital in the Philippines illustrating fast rotation among three 8-hour shifts, two 12-hour shifts, and 1 to 2 rest days per week (P. V. Bucalon, RN, oral communication, July 2021). (*B*) Sample 30-day schedule of a sleep technologist in the same private tertiary hospital showing slow rotation among two 8-hour evening shifts and one 8-hour morning shift (R. L. Legaspi, RMT, oral communication, July 2021).

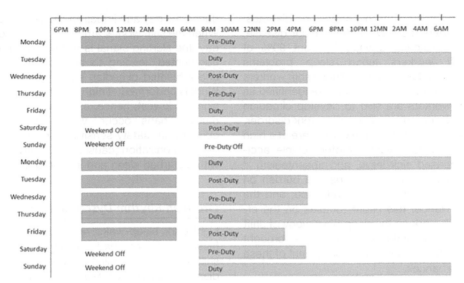

Fig. 3. Permanent or fixed schedule versus rotating schedule in shift workers. Green bars on the left show a sample 2-week schedule of a call center agent based in the Philippines who caters to US-based clients with a permanent or fixed 5-day 9-hour work week (B. A. Z. Pefianco, oral communication, July 2021). In contrast, orange bars on the right show a sample 2-week schedule of a surgical resident in a private tertiary hospital in the Philippines with a schedule that rotates among 3 early morning shifts: a 10-hour preduty shift, a 24-hour duty shift, and then a 10-hour postduty shift that immediately follows the duty shift (*Data from* St. Luke's Medical Center Department of ENT-HNS[6]).

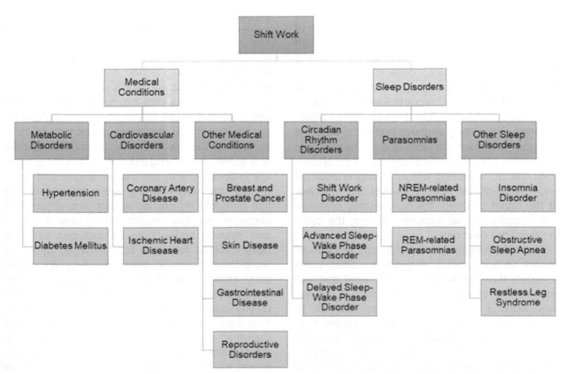

Fig. 4. Common medical comorbidities among shift workers. (*Data from* Keryezee[8], Khan[10], and Colten[11].)

consequences such as hypertension, diabetes, mood disorders, obesity, cardiovascular disease, and cerebrovascular disease.[11] About 90% of night shift workers report sleep problems compared with day workers.[12] Those shift workers who frequently change shifts and are identified as long-term workers are said to develop circadian system and sleep disruptions, shift work disorder, and social jet lag.[10] These individuals are at a high risk for workplace injuries, motor vehicle accidents, increased sick leave, and absenteeism.[13] The impact of these events poses a burden on the health care system, the workplace, and the economy. Hence, this paper focuses on the effects of shift work on the sleep physiology of shift workers, the different sleep disturbances brought about by shift work, and the management of these sleep disturbances.

SLEEP PHYSIOLOGY

Because of the nature of shift work, which entails individuals working during hours wherein sleep is normally expected, disruption of the circadian rhythm is often observed. The changes in sleep physiology can be explained by multiple factors, namely desynchronization of the two-process model of sleep regulation, disruption of the circadian rhythm, and an individual's morningness/eveningness or chronotype.

Two-Process Model of Sleep Regulation

The "two-process" model shows the interaction of homeostatic process (Process S) and circadian pacemaker (Process C).[14–16] In **Fig. 5**, Process S or the homeostatic sleep drive increases as we maintain wakefulness throughout the day. On the other hand, Process C is controlled by the suprachiasmatic nucleus (SCN), which facilitates wakefulness by increasing alertness during the day. The circadian pacemaker is facilitated by the rhythmic production and secretion of melatonin by attenuating the SCN alerting effect.[6] Sleep is attained once the peaks of both processes are reached. At the onset of sleep, the homeostatic pressure and circadian signal subside, allowing the cycle to repeat the next day.

Desynchronization of the two-process model occurs because shift work requires a sleep-wake schedule that conflicts with the natural endogenous rhythm of sleep and wakefulness.[16] Individuals working a night shift would attempt to initiate sleep during the time when Process C is elevated as seen in **Fig. 6**. They would then start their shift during the time when Process C is low. This forced disruption between sleep and activity patterns may explain the difficulty initiating sleep

during the day and impaired performance at night. When the shift worker attempts to sleep during the day, the alerting signal is highest; sleep becomes fragmented, leading to homeostatic sleep debt and a blunted circadian alerting system at night. Work is performed at night when circadian alerting signal is lowest; hence, excessive sleepiness and multiple naps occur, which are a particular concern in safety-sensitive environments. The desynchronization causes morbidity associated with disturbed sleep and impaired alertness.[4]

Circadian Rhythm Dysregulation

Light-dark, sleep-wake, rest-activity, and feeding-fasting cycles are inadvertently displaced among shift workers, increasing the likelihood of the circadian misalignment.[8] Sleep is being attempted when the level of melatonin is at its nadir, whereas work is performed when the level of melatonin is at its peak. Because the circadian rhythm is synchronized to daytime work and nighttime sleep, shift work would require phase adjustment, disrupting the normal organization and synchronization of the clock gene.[10] Disruption of the circadian clock by shift work alters important gene expression, leading to the suppression of core clock genes, such as *Per1*, *Per2*, and *MT1* melatonin, which causes further delays in the circadian acrophase.

Chronotype

The mechanisms behind the ability to sustain wakefulness during night shift and obtain substantial amount of sleep during nonworking times are poorly understood. Individual differences in tolerance to shift work may be due to differences in one's internal clock (chronotype).[16,17] "Morningness/eveningness" describes a trait that refers to the time of the day an individual is mostly awake and active.[15] "Morning larks" or early chronotypes are individuals who are mostly awake and functional in the early morning hours. "Night owls" or late chronotypes are individuals who experience alertness and functionality during late afternoon and evening hours. Late chronotypes seem to have a higher tolerance to shift work, with their work-sleep behavior seemingly less rigid than early chronotypes. They accumulate less sleep deficit during a shift work cycle and have better quality daytime sleep. As expected, however, they have more difficulties in early morning shifts than their early counterparts.[17] The differences in adaptability are also related to genetic polymorphism, melatonin profiles, and dim-light melatonin onset.[16]

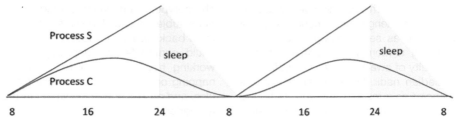

Fig. 5. Two-process model of sleep regulation. The Process S or the homeostatic sleep drive increases as wakefulness is maintained throughout the day. The Process C or the circadian pacemaker facilitates alertness during the day. (*Adapted from* Borbely[14], with permission.)

CHANGES IN SLEEP ARCHITECTURE
Shift Worker vs Nonshift Worker

When compared with nonshift workers, shift workers twice as often get less than 7 hours of nightly sleep during workdays, and 7 times as often get more than 9 hours of sleep during off-work days.[7] These differences were observed among those with morning chronotypes and advancing age. There is also a 4-hour difference in social jet lag between shift workers and nonshift workers in the older population. Other studies have found no difference in sleep duration between shift workers and nonshift workers, owing to the tendency of shift workers to sleep longer during transition to another shift and on off days. Chronotype may also influence a shift worker's sleep duration. Morning chronotype shift workers had a tendency to sleep short on work days and long on off days compared with nonshift workers. Shift workers with morning chronotypes tend to sleep shorter than a nonshift worker while on a night shift, a characteristic not observed among those with evening chronotypes.

Shift Work and Chronotype

Shift schedule and chronotype influence specific sleep characteristics of shift workers.[18] Individuals who are categorized as early chronotype sleep an hour earlier on a morning shift compared with those categorized as late chronotype who seem to have a higher tolerance to shift work.[17] Those with late chronotype tend to wake up late after a night shift and would have difficulty with early morning shifts.[17] Sleep duration was longer for early chronotypes on a morning shift and late chronotypes on an evening shift.

SLEEP DISTURBANCES

Circadian rhythm disturbances and sleep physiology changes that occur as a result of shift work will manifest as excessive sleepiness, difficulty sleeping, sleep deprivation, and social jet lag. Consequences of sleep disturbances influence mortality, morbidity, performance, accidents and injuries, functionality and quality of life, family and well-being, and health care utilization.[11]

Excessive Sleepiness

Postshift sleepiness, aside from insomnia, is the most common complaint of shift workers.[4] Epworth Sleepiness Scale (ESS) score of more than 10 was observed among 12.4% and ESS score of more than 16 in 2.9% both in men and women.[19] Men aged 45 to 54 years exhibited highest rate of sleepiness based on age group. Because of increased subjective and objective sleepiness, night shift workers would have involuntary sleep during early morning. This sleepiness is due to waking up at the nadir of the circadian pattern, wherein alertness is lowest and the need

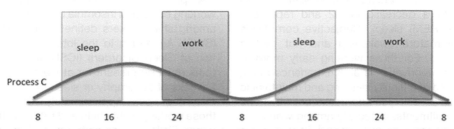

Fig. 6. Circadian misalignment. The purple line shows the Process C or the circadian activation. The blue boxes are the time shift workers on a night shift attempt to sleep during the say. The red boxes are the time of work. (*Data from* Kervezee[8], Khan[10], and Wickwire[16].)

for sleep is at its peak. This can also be caused by reduced prior sleep length and accumulation of sleep deprivation, as seen among chronic shift workers.[4] During a morning shift, there is pronounced difficulty of awakening, as this coincides with the circadian nadir. Nonrestorative sleep is also experienced as a result of the anticipation to wake up early, which causes decrease in slow wave sleep.

Difficulty Sleeping

Shift workers significantly experience difficulty initiating and maintaining sleep and early awakenings.[20] The desire to get enough sleep after a night shift results in an attempt to sleep earlier than the usual bedtime before the shift. This causes difficulty in sleep initiation due to its proximity to the circadian acrophase.[8,19] These symptoms may persist even after reverting back to conventional bedtimes, and this can be related to the partial adjustment of the circadian rhythm to the shift work schedule.[20] Around 15% to 20% of shift workers are health care professionals, and these individuals are exposed to traumatic situations that cause high levels of stress.[13] These situations can exacerbate sleep-related impairments, such as difficulty sleeping.

Sleep Deprivation

When sleep is displaced, the endogenous circadian pacemaker is disrupted, resulting in poor sleep quality and sleep deprivation.[21] Around 30% workers of nonstandard work schedules report sleeping less than 6 hours per day.[8] Severe sleep debt, defined as greater than 90 minutes decrease in sleep compared with baseline, was equally observed among 5% to 6% of men and women. For night shift workers, sleep is 2 to 4 hours less during bedtime and compensated by afternoon naps of more than 1 hour. Sleep is highest on the day before the first night shift and the day after the last night shift.[19] Around 55% of shift workers take a nap before the first night shift and 88% take a nap after the last night shift. Electroencephalogram patterns among shift workers demonstrate a decrease in N2 and rapid eye movement (REM) sleep.[7] Subjective complaints include premature awakening and not getting enough sleep. For those working early morning shifts, sleep deprivation is also experienced as a consequence of difficulty initiating and maintaining early bedtime.[6] Everyday domestic activities and social commitments, especially among women,[13] are likely to compete with sleep.[4] Shift workers stay awake longer, producing further accumulation of sleep debt. Regardless of the individual's

chronotype, sleep was observed to be shorter for older subjects, and sleep was longer for those doing a backward shift rotation.[18] Other factors that could contribute to sleep deprivation are long working hours, reduced rest periods, reduced napping opportunities, backward-rotating schedules, and on-call duties, on which further research is needed.[8]

Social Jet Lag

Social jet lag is defined as a shift in schedule between workdays and off days wherein sleep is longer during off days compared with workdays. Social jet lag, which is a key player in developing metabolic syndrome, is commonly observed among those with a late chronotype.[4] Around a 4.2-hour-per-day difference has been observed among shift workers compared with nonshift workers.[7] For shift workers, social jet lag is lower before, between, and after night shifts than before transitioning to a day shift. Social jet lag was highest with those doing night shift regardless of their chronotype.[18] Sleep need was found to be decreased to 7% between night shifts but increased to 15% the day before night shift, and 26% after the last night shift.[7]

SLEEP DISORDERS

Because of the rotating shifts that directly affect the light/d rhythm, different sleep disorders are commonly observed among shift workers.[10] Sleep disorders observed among long-term shift workers and those continuously changing shifts are seen in **Fig. 1**. Major sleep disorders are shift work disorder, jet lag disorder or social jet lag, and sleep disorders due to the disruption of the circadian system.

Circadian Rhythm Disorders

Because dysregulation of the circadian rhythm is the core problem among shift workers, there is a high risk of developing circadian rhythm disorders.

Shift work sleep disorder
The presence of excessive sleepiness during working hours and insomnia during sleep schedule among shift workers defines shift work disorder (SWD). According to the International Classification of Sleep Disorders (ICSD-3)[22], these symptoms must be present for at least 3 months, with 2 weeks of actigraphy or sleep log demonstrating disturbed sleep. Approximately 10% to 30%[8] of those working night shifts and rotating shifts experience SWD,[23] when shift workers' internal circadian rhythms are unable to adapt to shift schedules.[4] As high as 9% suffer from severe

SWD.[10] Older individuals and women were at higher risk for developing SWD. For the older age group, this may be due to the age-related changes in the homeostatic sleep drive and circadian signaling. Although less clear for women, risk for SWD could be due to sex-related differences in sleep, job assignment, and expected roles on going home.[15] Those who develop shift work disorder were noted to have shorter sleep duration, shorter sleep onset latency on multiple sleep latency test, hyperactivity to novel stimuli, and reduced brain response to auditory stimuli.[23]

Sleep-wake phase disorders

Advanced sleep-wake phase disorder (ASWPD) occurs when an individual's sleeping and waking times advance by 3 to 4 hours compared with the normal population.[10] An individual with delayed sleep-wake phase disorder (DSWPD), on the other hand, would have difficulty sleeping and arising during normal times due to delays in sleep timing. Because shift work has a direct impact on sleep, this may affect the normal functioning of the genes directly responsible for sleep, which may cause either ASWPD or DSWPD.

Other Sleep Disorders

Insomnia

Insomnia is the most commonly reported sleep disorder.[11] Around 10% of adults in the United States suffer from insomnia, and as high as 30% to 40% report symptoms of insomnia not fulfilling the ICSD-3 diagnostic criteria.[11,23,24] Insomnia is defined as difficulty initiating sleep, difficulty maintaining sleep, and early morning awakening despite adequate opportunity to sleep. The difficulty in sleeping causes multiple symptoms such as fatigue, cognitive impairment, mood disturbance, behavior problems, and excessive daytime sleepiness.[22] Shift workers have a higher prevalence of insomnia.[25] Chronic insomnia was experienced by 26.2% of shift workers, mostly among women aged 45 to 54 years.[19] Among those on rotating shifts, as high as 45% suffered from insomnia.[20] The nature of occupation, strenuous physical exertion, and continuous mental stress in the workplace were identified as risk factors for developing insomnia.[20] Shift workers tend to display depressed mood and low energy, which impair their quality of life and produce low-quality output in the workplace.[25] In the worst conditions, insomnia may increase workplace injuries and accidents.[24] Disturbed sleep, insomnia in particular, may promote comorbidity due to its presence across different conditions. As such, a chronic shift worker may be sensitized toward a transdiagnostic process of insomnia that may in turn worsen comorbid disorders.[7]

Sleep-related breathing disorders (obstructive sleep apnea)

The most common sleep-related breathing disorder is obstructive sleep apnea (OSA), with around 4% of men and 2% of women suffering from this disorder.[11] In OSA, repeated upper airway collapse occurs during sleep, causing significant oxygen desaturations and reduction in breathing amplitude called apneas and hypopneas. Polysomnography (PSG) that demonstrates an apnea-hypopnea index (AHI) of more than 5 with symptoms of excessive sleepiness, choking episodes, and comorbid medical conditions, such as hypertension, diabetes, or mood disorders, would diagnose a patient to have OSA. In the absence of symptoms, an AHI of 15 is required for a diagnosis of OSA.[22] Shift workers with OSA were noted to have increased AHI and more severe oxygen desaturations during PSG done during the daytime after an evening shift compared with a PSG done at night.[26] This could be due to the high occurrence of respiratory events during REM sleep, which manifests more during sleep in the biological morning.[27] Worsening of AHI for night shift workers places them at greater risk for hypertension, cardiovascular disease, impaired glucose tolerance, and obesity—all of which are identified as comorbidities of individuals with OSA.[11]

Sleep-related movement disorders (restless legs syndrome)

A common sleep-related movement disorder is restless legs syndrome (RLS), which is characterized as an unpleasant sensation on the legs experienced at night or during sedentary activities during the day. This unpleasant sensation can only be relieved on constant movement of the legs.[22] Around 26.8% of nurses working on shifts were noted to have RLS, which is higher than the general population.[12] Nurses who had SWD reported more RLS.[11] The symptoms are clearly circadian-related, because the unpleasant sensation is experienced at night and during transition from wake to sleep. Although studies show inconsistent results on the effect of shift work on chronic disruption of the circadian rhythm on RLS, chronic sleep deprivation and fatigue, which are common among shift workers, are said to trigger symptoms of RLS.

Parasomnia

Parasomnias are undesirable events or experiences that occur during either non-REM (NREM) or REM sleep. As listed in the ICSD-3, NREM-related parasomnias include confusional arousals, sleep or night terrors, sleepwalking (somnambulism), and sleep-related eating disorder; REM-related parasomnias include REM sleep behavior disorder, nightmare disorder, and recurrent isolated sleep paralysis.[22] There is a higher incidence of confusional arousals among night shift workers than day shift workers because increased sleep pressure is assumed to be a risk factor for developing NREM parasomnias. When there is increased sleep pressure, a rebound increase in slow wave sleep occurs in the first recovery night,[5] which increases the risk of developing confusional arousals among younger individuals.[28] There is also an increased risk of developing REM parasomnias, specifically nightmare disorder, due to the higher occurrence of REM sleep in daytime sleep; this is due to increased REM sleep propensity close to the nadir of core temperature.[28]

TREATMENT

A personalized treatment plan is ideal in the management of SWD,[16] which will involve tackling issues regarding circadian misalignment, sleepiness and sleep disturbances, and other special concerns (ie, safety).

Circadian Misalignment

As circadian misalignment seems to play a central role in the pathophysiology of shift work disorder,[5] it is sensible to target treatment approaches toward adjustment of or adaptation to this factor. Schedule alignment based on chronotype (ie, matching chronotype to shift time using the morningness-eveningness questionnaire or Munich chronotype questionnaire)[17] results in improved sleep duration and sleep quality and decrease in social jet lag.[18] Elimination of the shift work schedule is ideal but may be out of the question in most work settings. Bright light exposure (intermittent exposure to 3500–5000 lx)[17] 3 to 6 hours before the circadian nadir has been found to shift internal biological time,[21] which may help in circadian adaptation. The use of dark sunglasses when traveling home after shifts and of blackout curtains when indoors, on the other hand, may also provide shielding from light exposure and create an optimal environment for inducing sleep. The efficacy of this therapy is challenged by difficulty maintaining consistent activity and sleep-wake schedules in shift workers. Administration of chronobiotic compounds such as melatonin, recommended at a dosage of 3 mg before bedtime,[29] is indicated in order to promote daytime sleep among shift workers. However, the

intake of melatonin does not improve alertness during the night shift.[18]

Sleepiness and Sleep Disturbances

Sleep disturbances and poor-quality sleep are key features of SWD. Maintaining good sleep hygiene is a key approach to improving sleep and preventing sleep loss.[16] Instructions include limiting intake of alcohol and caffeinated products, obtaining regular moderate exercise, and maintaining a quiet and comfortable bedroom environment. Sleep anchoring—establishing a sleep period that overlaps on both work and non-workdays—creates a balance for shift workers to maintain personal and social routines while stabilizing their rhythms during workdays. Planned napping, including pre-shift sleep periods, can also increase total sleep time on top of improving alertness and vigilance.[29] Hypnotic medications, such as benzodiazepine (eg, triazolam) and nonbenzodiazepine agents (eg, zolpidem) may also be used to promote daytime sleep. It is important, however, to consider carryover effect of sedation to the shift work hours, which may pose adverse effects on work performance and safety.[18] Worsening of possible comorbid sleep conditions must also be considered.

Safety and Work Performance

Because of the potentially irregular nature of the sleep-wake in shift workers, safety is a major area of concern. Planned strategic napping for 1 to 1.5 hours, including early preshift sleep periods, increases alertness and vigilance and decreases accidents during work, without affecting postshift daytime sleep.[18,29] Psychostimulants such as modafinil, caffeine, and methamphetamine have been shown to enhance alertness, counter sleepiness, and improve psychomotor performance. Modafinil and caffeine have established safety records and therefore may be used when enhanced alertness is necessary. Combining measures such as preshift napping with other coping mechanisms such as caffeine intake (250–300 mg)[30] or bright light exposure[31] may also improve postshift alertness and performance.

SUMMARY

In order to meet the demands of a fast-growing economy, the need to perform specific tasks during nontraditional working hours has led to the evolution of shift work. Schedules for shift work remain varied: some shift workers maintain a morning, night, or evening shift but most will be following either forward or backward rotating shifts, with either fast or slow transitions.[3] When shift workers work at night and sleep during the day, the circadian rhythm is disrupted.[10] Circadian misalignment[16] is just one of the factors involved in the development of metabolic and cardiovascular health problems.[8] Aside from medical conditions[9] sleep disturbances, such as excessive sleepiness, insomnia, sleep deprivation, and social jet lag,[16] are also very evident in this population. Sleep disturbances are mostly experienced by women and those of older age,[4,16] and this may be due to the increase in occurrence of sleep disorders among these populations. These sleep disturbances eventually lead to circadian disorders and other sleep disorders.[10] Shift work disorder and other sleep-related impairments among shift workers vary between individuals despite similar schedules.[12] OSA,[26] RLS,[12] and NREM parasomnias[28] are worsened in night shift workers attempting sleep during the day. In spite of multiple effective suggested interventions, most shift workers find it difficult to comply with these behavioral modifications because these interventions offer only transient improvements in sleep.[18] Given the consequences of shift work on sleep, other than prevention and treatment guidelines, there is a need for comprehensive evaluation of those individuals who need to be awake during the night and asleep during the day.

CLINICS CARE POINTS

- Shift workers are potentially at risk for a variety of health problems due to the disturbance in the sleep physiology, which include metabolic syndrome, cardiovascular disease, and sleep disorders.

- The changes in sleep physiology are due to desynchronization of the two-process model of sleep regulation, disruption of the circadian rhythm, and mismatch of work schedule with individual's morningness/eveningness or chronotype.

- Evaluation for sleep disturbances among shift workers should involve the assessment of symptoms of excessive sleepiness, difficulty sleeping, sleep deprivation, and social jet lag. Screening for circadian rhythm disorders, sleep-related breathing disorders, sleep-related movement disorders, and parasomnias must be performed.

- Individuation of treatment is important for shift workers. Specific therapies must be used to target circadian misalignment, sleepiness and sleep disturbances, as well as safety and work performance. A combination of schedule alignment, sleep anchoring, planned strategic napping, timed bright light exposure, and administration of chronobiotic compounds such as melatonin is typically recommended.

- The use of hypnotic medications in order to promote daytime sleep should be done with caution, considering the carryover effect of sedation to shift work hours, as well as the presence of any comorbid conditions. Psychostimulants may be used when enhanced alertness is necessary.

DISCLOSURE

The authors have nothing to disclose.

REFERENCES

1. Parent-Thirion A, Vermeylen G, Cabrita J, et al. 6th European working conditions survey - overview report. Luxembourg: Publications Office of the European Union; 2017. Available at: https://www.eurofound.europa.eu/publications/report/2016/working-conditions/sixth-european-working-conditions-survey-overview-report. Accessed May 15, 2021.
2. U.S. Bureau of Labor Statistics. Job flexibilities and work schedules summary. Washington, DC: US Bureau of Labor Statistics; 2019. Available at: https://www.bls.gov/news.release/flex2.nr0.htm. Accessed May 17, 2021.
3. Redeker NS, Caruso CC, Hashmi SD, et al. Workplace interventions to promote sleep health and an alert, healthy workforce. J Clin Sleep Med 2019; 15(4):649–57.
4. Drake CL, Wright KP Jr. Shift work, shift-work disorder, and jet lag. In: Kryger MH, Roth T, Dement WC, editors. Principles and practice of sleep medicine. 6th edition. Philadelphia (PA): Elsevier; 2015. p. 714–25.
5. Lozano-Kühne J, Aguila M, Chua RB, et al. Shift work research in the Philippines: current state and future directions. Philippine Sci Lett 2012;5(1): 17–29.
6. Navarro-Locsin CG, Lim WL, et al. St. Luke's Medical Center Department of ENT-HNS. 2018-2019 Accreditation Report. Quezon City (Philippines): St. Luke's Medical Center; 2019.
7. Hulsegge G, Loef B, van Kerkhof LW, et al. Shift work, sleep disturbances and social jetlag in healthcare workers. J Sleep Res 2019;28(4):e12802.
8. Kervezee L, Kosmadopoulos A, Boivin DB. Metabolic and cardiovascular consequences of shift

work: the role of circadian disruption and sleep disturbances. Eur J Neurosci 2018;51(1):396–412.

9. Lu F, Suggs A, Ezaldein H, et al. The effect of shift work and poor sleep on self-reported skin conditions: a Survey of call center agents in the Philippines. Clocks Sleep 2019;1(2):273–9.

10. Khan S, Duan P, Yao L, et al. Shiftwork-mediated disruptions of circadian rhythms and sleep homeostasis cause serious health problems. Int J Genomics 2018;2018:1–11.

11.. Colten HR, Altevogt BM, Institute of Medicine (US). Committee on Sleep Medicine and Research. In: Colten HR, Altevogt BM, et al, editors. Sleep disorders and sleep deprivation: an unmet public health problem. Washington, DC: National Academies Press (US); 2006 p. 20–1. Available at: https://www.ncbi.nlm.nih.gov/books/NBK19960. Accessed May 17, 2021.

12. Waage S, Pallesen S, Moen BE, et al. Restless legs syndrome/willis-ekbom disease is prevalent in working nurses, but seems not to be associated with shift work schedules. Front Neurol 2018;9:21.

13. Booker LA, Magee M, Rajaratnam SMW, et al. Individual vulnerability to insomnia, excessive sleepiness and shift work disorder amongst healthcare shift workers. A systematic review. Sleep Med Rev 2018;41:220–33.

14. Borbély AA. A two process model of sleep regulation. Hum Neurobiol 1982;1(3):195–204.

15. Borbély AA, Daan S, Wirz-Justice A, et al. The two-process model of sleep regulation: a reappraisal. J Sleep Res 2016;25(2):131–43.

16. Wickwire EM, Geiger-Brown J, Scharf SM, et al. Shift work and shift work sleep disorder: clinical and organizational perspectives. Chest 2017;151(5): 1156–72.

17. Kantermann T, Juda M, Vetter C, et al. Shift-work research: where do we stand, where should we go? Sleep Biol Rhythms 2010;8(2):95–105.

18. Juda M, Vetter C, Roenneberg T. Chronotype modulates sleep duration, sleep quality, and social jet lag in shift-workers. J Biol Rhythms 2013;28(2):141–51.

19. Akerstedt T. Shift work and disturbed sleep/wakefulness. Occup Med (Lond) 2003;53(2):89–94.

20. Chatterjee K, Ambekar P. Study of insomnia in rotating shift-workers. Ind Psychiatry J 2017;26(1): 82–5.

21. Boivin DB, James FO. Light treatment and circadian adaptation to shift work. Ind Health 2005;43(1): 34–48.

22. American Academy of Sleep Medicine. The International Classification of Sleep Disorders. 3rd edition. Darien, IL: American Academy of Sleep Medicine; 2014.

23. Drake CL, Roehrs T, Richardson G, et al. Shift work sleep disorder: prevalence and consequences beyond that of symptomatic day workers. Sleep 2004;27(8):1453–62.

24. Jehan S, Zizi F, Pandi-Perumal SR, et al. Shift work and sleep: medical implications and management. Sleep Med Disord 2017;1(2):00008.

25. Dopheide JA. Insomnia overview: epidemiology, pathophysiology, diagnosis and monitoring, and nonpharmacologic therapy. Am J Manag Care 2020;26(4 Suppl):S76–84.

26. Paciorek M, Korczyński P, Bielicki P, et al. Obstructive sleep apnea in shift workers. Sleep Med 2011; 12(3):274–7.

27. Reid KJ, Abbott SM. Jet lag and shift work disorder. Sleep Med Clin 2015;10(4):523–35.

28. Bjorvatn B, Magerøy N, Moen BE, et al. Parasomnias are more frequent in shift workers than in day workers. Chronobiol Int 2015;32(10):1352–8.

29. Morgenthaler TI, Lee-Chiong T, Alessi C, et al. Practice parameters for the clinical evaluation and treatment of circadian rhythm sleep disorders. Sleep 2007;30(11):1445–59. An American Academy of Sleep Medicine report [Erratum appears in Sleep 2008; 31(7)].

30. Schweitzer PK, Randazzo AC, Stone K, et al. Laboratory and field studies of naps and caffeine as practical countermeasures for sleep-wake problems associated with night work. Sleep 2006;29(1):39–50.

31. Leger D, Philip P, Jarriault P, et al. Effects of a combination of napping and bright light pulses on shift workers' sleepiness at the wheel: a pilot study. J Sleep Res 2009;18(4):472–9.

Sleep Disturbance in Pregnancy

Somprasong Liamsombut, MD[a,b], Visasiri Tantrakul, MD[b,c],*

KEYWORDS

- Sleep disturbances • Sleep complaints • Pregnancy

KEY POINTS

- During pregnancy, alteration of sleep occurs related to the anatomic and physiologic changes in gestation.
- Sleep disturbances are common in pregnant women and can be due to the changes in pregnancy and/or the existing or aggravated sleep disorders.
- Poor sleep quality, insufficient sleep, and sleep disorders particularly obstructive sleep apnea contribute to adverse maternal and fetal outcomes.
- Screening and treatment of sleep disorders are important and may improve pregnancy outcomes.
- Promoting good sleep for healthy pregnancy should be integrated into routine antenatal care.

INTRODUCTION

Pregnancy is a vulnerable time for both the mother and fetus. Sleep as part of body and mind restoration plays an important role in maternal and fetal health. Inevitably, alteration in sleep occurred continuously throughout pregnancy due to the physiologic and hormonal changes.[1,2] Moreover, sleep disorder such as obstructive sleep apnea (OSA) can be aggravated or developed during this time.[3] Evidence had shown that OSA leads to several adverse outcomes including preeclampsia, gestational hypertension, gestational diabetes, preterm delivery, and stillbirth.[4] Short sleep duration and poor sleep quality could also lead to perinatal depression and gestational diabetes.[5,6] Socioeconomic status may contribute to the sleep loss in pregnant women as the mother's sleep is not protected.[7–9]

SLEEP CHANGES DURING PREGNANCY

Hormonal and physical changes in pregnancy cause alterations in sleep duration and architecture.[1,2] Total sleep time increases during the 1st trimester than nonpregnant period, thereafter it progressively decreases and is significantly reduced toward the 3rd trimester.[1,2] Deep sleep and REM sleep are reduced after the 1st trimester.[1,2] However, preeclamptic women had higher slow wave sleep than normal pregnant women (43 ± 3 vs $21 \pm 2\%, P < .001$).[10] Possible explanations for the increase in slow wave sleep might be related to cerebral edema and cytokine release (ie, tumor necrosis factor-α, interleukin-6, IL-6, and interleukin-8, IL-8) associated with preeclampsia.[10,11] Subjective perception of poor sleep quality was highly reported during the 3rd trimester in association with the changes in sleep macrostructure.[12] Izci -Balserak, et al. studied the changes in sleep architecture and EEG spectral analysis during early and late pregnancy.[13] It showed that pregnant women had shorter sleep duration, poorer sleep efficiency, more awakening, and higher N2 sleep with less slow wave and REM sleep, compared to nonpregnant counterpart.[13] Additionally, these changes subsequently worsened from early to late pregnancy.[13]

[a] Division of Pulmonary and Critical Care, Department of Medicine, Ramathibodi Hospital, Mahidol University, Bangkok, Thailand; [b] Division of Sleep Medicine, Department of Medicine, Ramathibodi Hospital, Mahidol University, Rama VI Road, Rachatevi, Bangkok 10400, Thailand; [c] Ramathibodi Hospital Sleep Disorder Center, Mahidol University, Bangkok, Thailand
* Corresponding author: Division of Sleep Medicine, Department of Medicine, Faculty of Medicine, Ramathibodi Hospital, Mahidol University, Rama VI Road, Rachatevi, Bangkok 10400, Thailand.
E-mail address: vtantrakul@gmail.com

Sleep Med Clin 17 (2022) 11–23
https://doi.org/10.1016/j.jsmc.2021.10.002
1556-407X/22/© 2021 Elsevier Inc. All rights reserved.

SLEEP COMPLAINTS DURING PREGNANCY
Common Sleep Complaints During Pregnancy

Most - pregnant women encounter at least 1 sleep problem especially towards the last trimester.[1,14] There are increasing reports that as pregnancy progresses, these common sleep complaints may overlap with symptoms of possible coexisting sleep disorders.[15] It is crucial to recognize and differentiate whether sleep complaints occur from pregnancy itself or a manifestation of a sleep disorder during pregnancy. This approach will improve their sleep quantity and quality and may improve pregnancy outcomes, see **Fig. 1**.

Excessive Daytime Sleepiness

Excessive daytime sleepiness (EDS) is common and may occur as the first sign of pregnancy.[16] EDS based on Epworth Sleepiness Scale (ESS) of more than 10 were reported in 32.1% to 45.5% of pregnant women.[15,16] Causes of EDS during pregnancy may be related to various factors, **Box 1**. The increase in total sleep time or frequent daytime naps during the 1st trimester is likely due to the alterations of hormonal levels such as progesterone, estrogen, prolactin, and oxytocin.[14,16,17] Sleep disruptions related to pregnant conditions such as frequent nocturia, discomfort from the gravid uterus, uterine contractions, musculoskeletal changes, fetal movements, and reflux symptoms may also contribute to EDS.[18] Additionally, chronic sleep insufficiency comprises a significant cause of EDS, with 29% of pregnant women reported shorter sleep duration (<6 hours/night).[17,18] Pregnant women were more likely to have sleep deprivation (odds ratio (OR): 3.9, 95% confidence interval (CI): 2.96, 5.16) than nonpregnant counterparts.[17] ESS scores significantly increased with the increasing gestational age (GA) from 1st to 3rd trimesters with a mean of 8.6 to 10.2, $P = .0003$.[15] Pregnant women who work nightshift were sleepier than those who work only during daytime.[18] The presence of EDS (ESS≥10) during the 3rd trimester

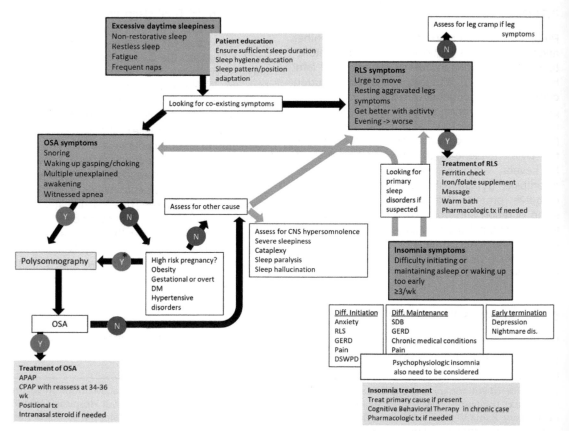

Fig. 1. Common manifestations of sleep disorders during pregnancy Y* Polysomnography may be considered in high-risk pregnant women who had daytime sleepiness despite adequate sleep and adaptation to physiologic changes during pregnancy. APAP, auto adjusting-continuous positive airway pressure therapy; CNS, central nervous system; CPAP, continuous positive airway pressure therapy; Diff., difficulty at; N, no; OSA, obstructive sleep apnea; RLS, restless legs syndrome; Y, yes.

Box 1
Causes of excessive daytime sleepiness during pregnancy

Causes of EDS* during the pregnancy

1. Hormonal changes

2. Sleep disruptions due to pregnancy conditions (eg, frequent nocturia, discomfort from the gravid uterus and musculoskeletal changes, uterine contractions, fetal movements, and gastrointestinal reflux)

3. Chronic sleep deprivation (<6 hours)

4. Coexisting sleep disorders worsen during pregnancy (eg, obstructive sleep apnea, restless leg syndrome, periodic limb movements)

5. Unrelated sleep disorders

Abbreviation: EDS* excessive daytime sleepiness.

had been associated with being employed, increasing arm circumference, and neonatal weight.[19]

However, the EDS may not be solely due to the normal changes of pregnancy.[20] Pathologic sleep disorders that are aggravated during pregnancy may also cause sleep fragmentation and EDS. Among these includes OSA, restless leg syndrome (RLS), and periodic limb movements (PLMs).[21,22] Most of the pregnant women had ESS less than 10, 19% had ESS $\geq$ 10, and only 1.7% had ESS $\geq$ 16.[20] There is a correlation between the increasing score of ESS and other symptoms of OSA such as loud snoring, gasping, and choking/apnea.[20] Interestingly, the association between the increasing score of ESS and other symptoms of OSA and adverse pregnancy outcomes was not significant at the conventional cut-off of hypersomnolence (ESS > 10).[16,20] Study had shown that EDS (ESS > 10) was not associated with snoring and gestational hypertension/ diabetes.[16] However, high level of EDS (ESS > 16) was associated with gestational diabetes and other symptoms of OSA (loud snoring, gasping, choking/apnea).[20] Recent study had shown that pregnant women with ESS $\geq$ 11 were less likely to achieve a spontaneous vaginal delivery (adjusted OR: 0.43, 95% CI: 0.21, 0.88), increased use of instrumentation and cesarean section (adjusted OR: 2.32, 95% CI: 1.14, 4.71), and higher poor neonatal outcomes (adjusted OR: 2.77, 95% CI: 1.09, 7.03).[23]

Although EDS (ESS > 10) alone may not be discriminative for OSA during pregnancy, exploration of other coexisting symptoms and risk factors of OSA can be helpful.[24,25] For OSA, its hallmark symptom "snoring" should be looked for in pregnant women with EDS. The cardinal symptoms of RLS and the accompanying PLMs should also be investigated.[26] Although uncommon, other coexisting sleep disorders unrelated to pregnancy such as "narcolepsy" should also be explored. Data on narcolepsy in pregnancy are scarce. The prevalence probably is similar to that in nonpregnant population.[14]

SNORING

Snoring, a sign of increased upper airway resistance, usually coincides with the diagnosis of sleep disordered breathing (SDB) in pregnant women. The prevalence of snoring ranges from 14% to 48% in normal pregnant women and up to 70% in those with risks factors such as obesity, gestational diabetes, or pregnancy-related hypertensive disorders.[27,28] Snoring was reported in 14% of pregnancy, approximately 3 times higher than nonpregnant women.[29] Reports of snoring increased as pregnancy progressed from 7% in 1st trimester, 6% in 2nd trimester, and 24% in 3rd trimester.[30] Snoring rate during the 3rd trimester was higher than prepregnancy and postpartum period with a frequency of 59%, 12%, and 18%, respectively.[27,31] Furthermore, reports of snoring were highest among preeclamptic women (75%) than pregnant women (28%), and nonpregnant counterparts (14%), $P = .02$.[31] The upper airway dimension was narrower in preeclamptic women both in upright and supine positions than uncomplicated pregnant, and nonpregnant women.[27] Narrowing of upper airway in preeclamptic women leads to obstructive respiratory events which could cause increases in blood pressures.[32] Many studies had shown that frequent snoring (snoring $\geq$3 times/wk) was a predictor of OSA during pregnancy.[25,33] Although snoring is still the cardinal symptoms of OSA during pregnancy, other symptoms may be less predictive.[34,35] Complaints of EDS, frequent nocturnal awakening, and fatigue are also commonly reported as symptoms of pregnancy.[34,35] The Sleep Apnea Symptom Score (SASS), the symptomology-based score demonstrated less accuracy for OSA prediction during the 1st and 3rd trimesters with C-statistics of 0.72 (0.58, 0.86) and 0.57 (0.43, 0.71), respectively.[34,35] Furthermore, snoring had adverse pregnancy outcomes similar to OSA.[36] A meta-analysis showed that snoring alone was associated with pregnancy induced hypertension (OR: 1.80; 95% CI: 1.28, 2.52), preeclampsia (OR: 1.87; 95% CI: 1.27, 2.75), gestational diabetes (OR: 2.14; 95% CI:

1.63, 2.81), and preterm birth (OR: 1.22; 95% CI: 0.87, 1.70).[36]

INSOMNIA

Insomnia is a common sleep problem encountered in the general population and during pregnancy.[37] A meta-analysis indicated that 38.2% of pregnant women experienced insomnia symptoms defined as having dissatisfaction with sleep quantity or quality at least ≥3 times per week for at least 3 months.[37] The highest insomnia prevalence fell into the 3rd trimester with 42.4% of participants experiencing the symptoms.[38] Although insomnia symptoms may be due to the pregnancy-related discomforts, it can be a manifestation of various sleep disorders.[1,6]

Primary or psychophysiological insomnia consisted of maladaptive sleep behaviors and coping strategies such as napping, or spending more time in bed can also perpetuate insomnia.[14,19] Moreover, emotional factors including stress about a new child, lifestyle changes, motherhood-work balance, and/or labor and delivery that accumulated during gestation may influence insomnia by increasing cortical arousals.[37]

Secondary or comorbid insomnia with other sleep disorders may also contribute.[14] Patients with OSA may have sleep disruptions and present as having sleep maintenance insomnia, whereas patients with RLS may have prolonged sleep latency due to the "URGE" symptoms (**Box 2**).[26] Nocturnal gastroesophageal reflux disease (GERD) is another common condition during pregnancy that causes sleep difficulty.[39] Its high prevalence of 26% during the 1st trimester may double to 51% in the 3rd trimester due to the increased abdominal pressure and peak hormonal levels.[40]

Cognitive-behavioral therapy for insomnia may be indicated, particularly stimulus control and relaxation technique in both primary and secondary insomnia.[41] Pharmacological therapy with relatively safe profile such as nonbenzodiazepine receptor agonists (zaleplon, zolpidem, and eszopiclone) may be considered in severe refractory insomnia despite treating the primary cause.[41]

PARASOMNIA/ABNORMAL MOVEMENT DURING SLEEP

Data on parasomnia prevalence during pregnancy are lacking. Regardless of pregnancy status, the prevalence in this age group should be no more than 4%.[42] A surveillance study reported a decline of NREM parasomnia episodes in pregnant women.[43] Nevertheless, nightmare was reported to increase during the last trimester probably due

---

Box 2
Characteristics symptoms of restless legs syndrome

The "URGE"[82] acronym for diagnosis of RLS/ WED*

U	An Urge to move the legs usually accompanied or thought to be caused by uncomfortable and unpleasant sensations in the legs
R	Resting or inactive state precipitates or worsens the unpleasant sensation or the urge to move symptom.
G	Getting relieved partially or completely with active movement of affected limbs is observed as long as the activity continues.
E	During Evening or night, the urge or unpleasant sensations are worse than that during the day.

The symptoms mentioned above are not entirely contributed to another medical or a behavioral condition (eg, legs cramp, venous stasis, leg edema, or position discomfort) and cause concern, distress, sleep disturbance, or impairment of mental, physical, social, behavioral, or other important areas of functioning.

Abbreviation: RLS/WED*, Restless legs syndrome/Willis–Ekbom disease.

Data from Allen RP, Picchietti DL, Garcia-Borreguero D, et al. Restless legs syndrome/Willis–Ekbom disease diagnostic criteria: updated International Restless Legs Syndrome Study Group (IRLSSG) consensus criteria–history, rationale, description, and significance. Sleep Med. 2014;15(8):860-873.[82]

---

to increased stress and anxiety.[44] Furthermore, patients with RLS may present with legs movements during sleep which is typically found up to 80%.[45]

SLEEP DISORDERS DURING PREGNANCY
Obstructive Sleep Apnea

Alterations of the anatomy, physiology, and hormonal levels during pregnancy increase the risks for the development of OSA or exacerbation of the preexisting condition.[31] These include weight gain, a 20% decrease in functional residual capacity (FRC) due to the displacement of the diaphragm from gravid uterus which further results in decreased oxygenation from increases in alveolar-arterial gradient (A-a) O_2 and ventilation-perfusion mismatch.[46] Normal pregnancy is associated with progressive rightward shift of the oxyhemoglobin dissociation curve, which facilitates the oxygen off-loading to peripheral tissues and is beneficial to the placenta.[47] In contrast, a leftward shift of oxyhemoglobin dissociation curve is found in preeclampsia which impaired oxygen off-loading, rendering the fetus vulnerable to even subtle obstructive respiratory events.[47]

Narrowing of the upper airway and increase in the upper airway resistance in pregnant women particularly during the 3rd trimester may result from the nasopharyngeal and oropharyngeal edema from the increases in estrogen level and circulatory blood volume.[31,46] Additionally, sleep deprivation and fragmentation negatively affect pharyngeal muscle activity and upper airway collapsibility.[46] Rhinitis symptoms were commonly found during pregnancy due to the increase in estrogen level,[48] whereas the increase in progesterone level showed protective effect by up-regulating the ventilatory drive, and increasing the genioglossus dilator muscle activity.[48,49] Pregnant women with OSA demonstrated lower progesterone levels.[49]

The prevalence of OSA had increased over the past decades as obesity had risen in the population. Recently, the US National cohort of pregnancy from 2010 to 2014 showed the rate of OSA at 0.12%.[50] Based on home sleep apnea test (HSAT) with apnea–hypopnea index (AHI) $\geq$5 events/h, a cohort of normal pregnancy showed prevalence of OSA during 1st trimester and mid-pregnancy of 3.5% and 8.5% with the new-onset OSA during pregnancy of 5.8%.[33] However, the prevalence of OSA based on AHI $\geq$ 5 events/h from polysomnography (PSG) in high-risk pregnant women with obesity, and other risk factors (ie, chronic hypertension, history of preeclampsia, gestational diabetes, or twin gestation) were higher during the 1st and 3rd trimesters at 30% and 47%.[51] A study on Asian pregnant women with high-risk factors (ie, obesity, chronic hypertension, gestational diabetes, history of preeclampsia) showed a higher prevalence of OSA (AHI $\geq$ 5 events/h from Watch-PAT) during their 1st, 2nd, and 3rd trimesters at 30.4%, 33.3%, and 32.0%, respectively.[25] Variation in the prevalence of OSA during pregnancy may depend on several factors including population studied (high risk vs general pregnancy), ethnicity, trimesters, type of sleep testing (PSG vs HSAT), and the criteria of diagnosis (AHI vs respiratory disturbance index, RDI, and different hypopnea criteria).[52] A meta-analysis showed the overall pooled OSA prevalence during pregnancy of 15% (95% CI: 12%, 18%) with high heterogeneity $I^2 = 86.2\%$.[52] Their sensitivity

analyses showed variations among world regions (range 5%–20%), trimesters studied (range 11%–19%), and definition of hypopneas used (range 15%–24%).[52] Although highly prevalent, OSA during pregnancy is under-recognized among patient and provider.[53]

Accuracy of screening questionnaires showed poor discrimination of Berlin questionnaire and ESS ($\geq$10) and for OSA diagnosis in pregnant population.[25,54] A meta-analysis reported the pooled sensitivity and specificity (95% CI) of 0.66 (0.45, 0.83) and 0.62 (0.48, 0.75) for Berlin questionnaire.[24] Accuracy became less when used during early pregnancy (GA <20 weeks) and in high-risk pregnancy.[24] Study on obese parturient showed that STOP-Bang questionnaire of a higher score increased the probability of OSA from less than 10% for a score less than 3 to 68% with a score of 6. However, the predicted probability of having OSA was 5.0% for no snoring and 26.4% for snoring, indicating that snoring maybe a simpler and effective predictor of OSA.[55] Screening of OSA during pregnancy based on these questionnaires and/or self-reported symptoms alone may be less predictive because of the overlapping symptoms of OSA and pregnancy.[34,35]

Several prediction models specific for gestational OSA were developed including Facco, Iczi-Balserak (BATE: BMI, age, Tongue enlargement), Louis, and Wilson models, along with external validation of the Multivariable Apnea Prediction Questionnaire (MVAP), a general prediction model for OSA.[33,34,56,57] These models showed better performances than questionnaires with pooled c-statistics (95% CI) of 0.81 (0.783, 0.850) and 0.855 (0.822, 0.887) for the 1st, 2nd and 3rd trimesters OSA.[56] Only Facco and the MVAP models were externally validated. BMI, age, and snoring were the most common predictors among these models.[56,57] However, there is a limitation in the generalizability of these prediction models given the high heterogeneity between studies.[56] Nevertheless, these prediction models maybe helpful in guiding and prioritizing the need for further objective sleep test.

Diagnosis of gestational OSA by a gold standard type 1 PSG is challenging given the difficulty in access, the discomfort to the pregnant women, and the limited timing of pregnancy. Some HSAT had been used in pregnant women with more convenience.[58,59] Watch-PAT, a wrist-worn device using a peripheral arterial tonometry (PAT), finger plethysmography, and pulse oximeter, had been validated in pregnant women and showed good accuracy for gestational OSA based on AHI and RDI $\geq$ 5 events/h with C-statistics (95% CI) of 0.95 (0.88, 1.00) and 0.94 (0.86, 1.00), respectively.[59] Whereas the agreements for ApneaLink versus PSG for AHI $\geq$ 5 events/h in 2nd trimester obese pregnant women were 83.3% and 76.7% for auto and manual scorings.[58] Most of the OSA during pregnancy were in the mild range;[51] however, airflow limitation or partial airway obstruction had been shown to increase in pregnant women regardless of AHI.[51,60] However, subtle obstructive respiratory events such as respiratory-event related arousal (RERA) and airflow limitation were demonstrated to increase blood pressure level similar to that of apnea/hypopnea in the pregnant population.[61] Recently pulse-transit-time, a novel metrics for diagnosis of OSA during pregnancy had been proposed, which showed better correlation with airflow limitation and sympathetic activation than conventional AHI.[62]

The pathophysiological effects of OSA causing oxygen desaturation, arousals, sympathetic activation, and endothelial dysfunction[63,64] are associated with the development of preeclampsia, and possible abnormal placentation during early pregnancy,[65,66] see **Fig. 2**.

Continuous positive airway pressure (CPAP) is the standard treatment of OSA in nonpregnant population. Data on the efficacy of CPAP treatment in gestational OSA are limited despite its safety use.[67] CPAP also has been proposed as the adjunctive treatment of preeclampsia due to the increase in airflow limitation that occurred in conjunctions with the increases in nocturnal blood pressure, total peripheral vascular resistance (TPR), and reduction in cardiac output (CO) during sleep.[32,68]

Restless Legs Syndrome in Pregnancy

Restless legs syndrome (RLS), or Willis–Ekbom disease (WED), is commonly found in pregnant women. A meta-analysis reported the ethnic variations in RLS prevalence during pregnancy ranging from 14% in East Asia, 21% to 22% in European and American regions to 30% in Eastern Mediterranean countries.[69] The prevalence of RLS in Thai pregnant women was reported to be 11.2%.[70] RLS increases with gestation with estimated pooled prevalence during the 1st, 2nd, and 3rd trimesters of 8%, 16%, and 22%, respectively.[69]

Pathophysiology

Evidence had shown that patients with RLS had decreased iron metabolism in multiple brain regions including substantia nigra, red nucleus, thalamus, and striatum.[71,72] The iron depletion hypothesis seems to be valid even in pregnant women as supported by studies in East Asia.[73,74] Chen and colleagues found significant

associations of RLS in pregnancy with anemia, peptic ulcer disease, lower iron, and folate supplements.[73] However, other studies did not find associations between iron status and/or hemoglobin level and RLS in pregnant women.[75,76] Moreover, the rapid recovery of RLS symptoms after delivery might not be explained by this hypothesis as iron restoration is usually not completed by that time.[77] Another proposed pathogenesis of RLS during pregnancy involves hormonal changes. Increases in estradiol, progesterone, and prolactin levels, peaking in the 3rd trimester corresponded to the higher prevalence compared with early GA, may play a role.[78] Estradiol and progesterone levels dramatically decrease after delivery, when RLS usually disappears.[79] Genetic factor may also be substantial as family history of RLS was present in most of the pregnant women with RLS.[80] Additionally, women who developed RLS during pregnancy had a 4-fold higher risk of developing idiopathic RLS later on.[81]

Diagnosis of Restless Leg Syndrome

The diagnosis of RLS required a history of clinical presentations plus an exclusion of other possible conditions as recommended by the International Restless Legs Syndrome Study Group (IRLSSG).[26] The diagnostic criteria are simplified by the acronym "URGE"[26,82] represented in **Box 2**.

Despite using the same criteria with general population, the challenge of RLS diagnosis during pregnancy occurs because pregnancy-related conditions may mimic RLS symptoms. These conditions include leg cramp, positional discomfort, compression and stretched neuropathy, venous stasis, and legs edema. The unpleasant RLS symptoms may be underreported due to patient's misperception of symptoms as part of pregnancy-related changes.[26,82]

Treatment

RLS symptoms during pregnancy can manifest in a wide range of severity. Nonpharmacological treatment should be first considered given the less harmful effect to the fetus especially if sleep, mood, or quality of life is not significantly affected.[26]

Nonpharmacological Treatment

Avoidance of RLS aggravating factors is recommended such as sedating anti-histamines, anti-emetic dopaminergic antagonists, anti-depressant, caffeine, smoking, alcohol drinking, and sleep deprivation. Conditions that need to be addressed include iron deficiency anemia, prolonged immobilization,[83] coexisting sleep apnea, and peripheral

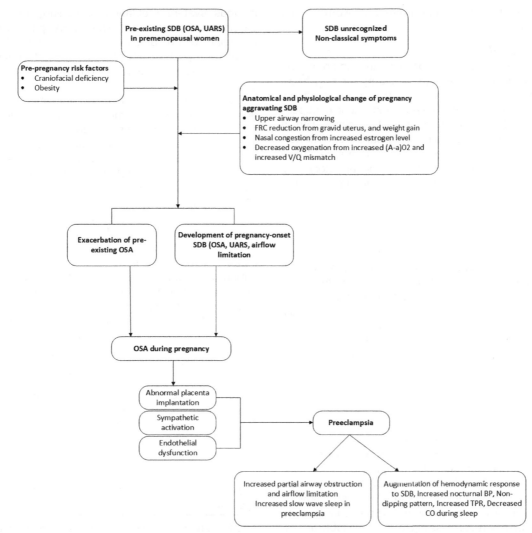

Fig. 2. The pathophysiological association linking obstructive sleep apnea and preeclampsia. (A-a) O_2, alveolar-arterial oxygen gradient; BP, blood pressure; CO, cardiac output, FRC, functional residual capacity; OSA, obstructive sleep apnea; SDB, sleep-disordered breathing; TPR, total peripheral resistance; UARS, upper airway resistance syndrome; V/Q mismatch, ventilation/perfusion mismatch.

neuropathy.[26] Moderate physical activity exercise such as yoga, water aerobics, or walking as well as warm/hot bath, legs massage, or pneumatic splinting may be beneficial to RLS.[83,84] Iron and folate supplementations as standard antenatal care are recommended. Ferritin and other iron status indicators should be assessed in pregnant women with RLS.[84] Ferritin level less than 75 µg/L should be a threshold to start or increase in iron supplement.[78] If serum ferritin is still less than 30 µg/L despite oral supplement, intravenous iron therapy will be indicative given its safety profile.[26]

Pharmacological Treatment

Pharmacological treatment should be considered for patients with persistent symptoms (≥2 times/

wk) and clinically severe RLS with International RLS severity rating scale greater than 20, despite proper nonpharmacological therapy.[78,85] Medication should be at the lowest effective level for the shortest duration while avoiding during the 1st trimester if possible.[78,80]

Dopamine agonist

Dopamine agonist is recognized as the first-line medication for RLS.[83,84] There was limited data supporting the use of pramipexole, ropinirole, and rotigotine in pregnancy, and thus the extended release form of carbidopa/levodopa at 25/100 to 50/200 µg/d in the evening might be more preferable.[26] Overall, there was no report of major fetal malformation in pregnant women using this medication.[86]

Alpha-2-delta-ligand

Gabapentin enacarbil, gabapentin, and pregabalin have gained increasing popularity for RLS treatment in general considering their positive effects and tolerant profile. However, high-dose gabapentin (400 mg/kg) intraperitoneal administration in mice was associated with impaired central nervous system synaptophysis.[87] Therefore, these drugs are limited to use only for refractory RLS treatment during lactation due to minimal drug secretion via breast milk.[88]

Benzodiazepine and benzodiazepine receptor agonist

Benzodiazepine and benzodiazepine receptor agonist are usually prescribed as adjunctive 2nd or 3rd line treatment of chronic idiopathic RLS. Additional effects to the 1st line treatment include facilitating and maintaining sleep, reducing arousal threshold, and controlling sensory legs symptoms.[78] Clonazepam seems to have no teratogenic risk and may be considered.[89] However, temazepam had been reported to associate with stillbirth when used in combination with diphenhydramine.[90]

Opioids

Opioids have been prescribed for the treatment of severe refractory RLS in general patients. However, opioid had demonstrated fetal malformation risks such as congenital heart disease, neural tube defects, and musculoskeletal malformations.[91] Therefore, opioids should not be prescribed during pregnancy regardless of GA.[92] If inevitably necessary, tramadol may be preferred due to its better safety profile than others in this category.[26]

CONSEQUENCES OF SLEEP DISTURBANCE ON MATERNAL AND FETAL OUTCOMES
Sleep Disturbance and Maternal and Fetal Consequences

Although strong evidence in general population had suggested associations between sleep disturbance with cardiovascular morbidity and mortality as well as impact on the quality of life, neurocognitive impairment, and motor vehicle accidents, less is known about the impact on maternal-fetal outcomes.[93]

Hypertensive Disorders of Pregnancy: Preeclampsia and Gestational Hypertension

Hypertensive disorder of pregnancy is a major contributor to maternal and fetal morbidity worldwide. Sleep state is vital to autonomic nervous system regulation particularly for the cardiovascular system.[94] The typical pattern of circadian blood pressure dipping (10%–20% drop in SBP) can be interfered by sleep disorders such as sleep restriction, sleep fragmentation, or SDB.[95]

Chronic sleep deprivation and sleep fragmentation from OSA causes sympathetic hyperactivity[96] and/or cortical arousals leading not only to nocturnal but also diurnal hypertension and long-term cardiovascular complications.[64] A meta-analysis had demonstrated the association of OSA and increased risk of gestational diabetes (OR: 1.71, 95% CI: 1.23, 2.38), preterm birth (OR: 1.75, 95% CI: 1.21, 2.55), preeclampsia (OR: 2.63, 95% CI: 1.87, 3.70), and pregnancy-induced hypertension (OR: 1.93, 95% CI: 1.63, 2.28).[36] A multistate large cohort with over 6.9 million participants reported that having OSA increased the risk of preeclampsia (OR: 2.05, 95% CI: 1.86, 2.29), pulmonary edema (OR: 4.73, 95% CI: 2.84, 7.89), and cesarean delivery (OR: 1.96, 95% CI: 1.81, 2.11).[50] Additionally, OSA during pregnancy was associated with 2.5 to 3.5-fold increase in the risk of severe complications such as cardiomyopathy, congestive heart failure, and hysterectomy. Length of hospital stay was significant longer (5.1 $\pm$ 5.6 vs 3.0 $\pm$ 3.0 days, $P < .001$) and higher intensive care unit admission (OR: 2.74, 95% CI: 2.36, 3.18).[50]

Hyperglycemia and Gestational Diabetes Mellitus

Accumulating evidence demonstrated an association between sleep disorders during pregnancy and hyperglycemia, although the causal relationship has not been firmly established.[14] During sleep, circadian-driven glucose metabolism occurs, mediating through hormonal regulations mainly insulin, cortisol, and growth hormone.[97] Sleep loss or disruption led to increased insulin resistance and hyperglycemia via multiple pathways such as increased sympathetic activity, increased systemic inflammatory response (ie, IL-1, IL-6, TNF-a, and C-reactive protein), and alterations of appetite-regulating hormones.[97] A meta-analysis estimated that pregnant women who slept $\leq$6.25 hours had higher 1-h glucose level after 50 g oral-glucose challenge test by 0.65 mmol/L (0.18–1.13) and an increased risk of GDM (adjusted OR: 2.84, 95% CI: 1.25, 6.44).[5] Another meta-analysis of 7 studies on patients with GDM found a significant association between GDM and OSA (adjusted OR: 1.53, 95% CI: 1.26, 1.9).[52]

Adverse Obstetric Outcomes

Sleep deprivation may lead to difficult delivery due to the inadequate physical and mental restoration from sleep during the 3rd trimester of pregnancy.[98] A large population-based cohort in Sweden studied 10,662 nulliparous women presenting with a singleton cephalic baby. Results showed that short sleep duration or sleep disturbance in the last trimester is an independent risk factor for emergency cesarean delivery (adjusted OR: 1.57, 95% CI: 1.14, 2.16).[99] OSA had also been shown to be associated with poor obstetric outcomes as reported in several studies.[21,50,52] Lui B et al. performed a 7-year cohort and reported that OSA was associated with poor obstetric outcomes such as cesarean section (adjusted OR: 1.96, 95% CI: 1.81, 2.11), and prolonged length of stay of more than 5 days (adjusted OR: 2.42, 95% CI: 2.21, 2.6).[50]

Fetal Adverse Outcomes

Fetal growth and development depend inevitably on maternal health and well-being. The peak secretion of growth hormone and uteroplacental blood flow occurs during maternal sleep;[100] therefore, poor maternal sleep or sleep disorders may alter uterine environment and adversely affect fetal formation and development.[101] Sleep restriction is a common problem found in working pregnant women. The similar increases in common inflammatory markers such as IL-1, IL-6, and IL-8 both in amniotic fluid of preterm labor mothers and the blood circulation of sleep-deprived pregnant women created an association hypothesis.[102] Micheli and colleagues demonstrated in their prospective cohort of greater than 10,000 nullipara that sleep-deprived mothers (defined as $\leq$5 hours per day) were at increased risk for preterm labor (adjusted OR: 1.7, 95% CI: 1.1, 2.8).[103] A meta-analysis showed that pregnant shift-workers had an increased risk of preterm delivery (relative risk (RR): 1.16, 95% CI: 1.00–1.33), and small for GA (RR: 1.12, 95% CI: 1.03, 1.22). However, most of the studies were small in sample size and some had significant methodological issue.[104]

There were accumulating data on the association of maternal SBD and poor fetal outcomes. Potential mechanisms include increased systemic inflammation, chronic intermittent hypoxemia of the fetus, uteroplacental dysfunction as well as consequences related to accompanying preeclampsia and GDM.[105]

A meta-analysis of 33 studies with more than 1 million participants reported that maternal SDB was associated with increases in preterm birth (OR: 1.86, 95% CI: 1.5, 2.31), low birth weight (OR: 1.67, 95% CI: 1.00–2.78), low APGAR score (<7) at 5 minute (OR: 2.14, 95% CI: 1.74, 3.71), stillbirth (OR: 2.02, 95% CI: 1.25, 3.28), and neonatal ICU admission (OR: 1.9, 95% CI: 1.38, 2.61).[106]

Maternal Psychosocial Outcomes

Pregnancy itself can be very stressful for expectant mothers. Antenatal depression is one of the major causes of disease burden and can be found as high as 15% to 65% of pregnant women worldwide.[107]

Sleep loss, sleep disruption, and SDB had been known to be associated with mood disorders.[108] Although not completely understood, the pathophysiology may involve the imbalance of monoaminergic-cholinergic neuron activity and the hypothalamic–pituitary adrenal regulations which can affect or be reflected through sleep duration and architecture.[108] Insomnia, whether through poor sleep quality or sleep loss, was strongly associated with depressive symptoms during late pregnancy particularly in those with sleep duration shorter than 5 hours a day.[109]

SUMMARY

Significant anatomic and physiologic changes occur during pregnancy leading to the alteration of sleep architecture. Sleep disturbances are common in pregnant women and can be both due to these changes and an existing or aggravated sleep disorders. Poor sleep quality, insufficient sleep, and sleep disorders contribute to adverse maternal and fetal outcomes. Screening and treatment of sleep disorders are important and may improve pregnancy outcomes. Sleep education should be given to both patients and careprovider to promote good sleep for healthy pregnancy and sleep care service should be integrated into routine antenatal care.

AUTHOR CONTRIBUTIONS

Conceptualization S. Liamsombut and V. Tantrakul; Writing- original draft, S. Liamsombut and V. Tantrakul; Writing-review& editing, S. Liamsombut and V. Tantrakul. All authors have read and agreed to the published version of the article.

DISCLOSURE

The authors have nothing to disclose.

REFERENCES

1. Lee KA, Zaffke ME, McEnany G. Parity and sleep patterns during and after pregnancy. Obstet Gynecol 2000;95(1):14–8.

2. Driver HS, Shapiro CM. A longitudinal study of sleep stages in young women during pregnancy and postpartum. Sleep 1992;15(5):449–53.

3. O'Brien LM, Bullough AS, Chames MC, et al. Hypertension, snoring, and obstructive sleep apnoea during pregnancy: a cohort study. BJOG 2014; 121(13):1685–93.

4. Pamidi S, Pinto LM, Marc I, et al. Maternal sleep-disordered breathing and adverse pregnancy outcomes: a systematic review and metaanalysis. Am J Obstet Gynecol 2014;210(1):52.e1–14.

5. Reutrakul S, Anothaisintawee T, Herring SJ, et al. Short sleep duration and hyperglycemia in pregnancy: aggregate and individual patient data meta-analysis. Sleep Med Rev 2018;40:31–42.

6. Okun ML, Kline CE, Roberts JM, et al. Prevalence of sleep deficiency in early gestation and its associations with stress and depressive symptoms. J Womens Health 2013;22(12):1028–37.

7. Christian LM, Carroll JE, Teti DM, et al. Maternal sleep in pregnancy and postpartum Part I: mental, physical, and interpersonal consequences. Curr Psychiatry Rep 2019;21(3):20.

8. Blair LM, Porter K, Leblebicioglu B, et al. Poor sleep quality and associated inflammation predict preterm birth: heightened risk among african Americans. Sleep 2015;38(8):1259–67.

9. Barazzetta M, Ghislandi S. Family income and material deprivation: do they matter for sleep quality and quantity in early life? Evidence from a longitudinal study. Sleep 2017;40(3):zsw066.

10. Edwards N, Blyton CM, Kesby GJ, et al. Preeclampsia is associated with marked alterations in sleep architecture. Sleep 2000;23(5):619–25.

11. Jonsson Y, Rubèr M, Matthiesen L, et al. Cytokine mapping of sera from women with preeclampsia and normal pregnancies. J Reprod Immunol 2006;70(1–2):83–91.

12. Garbazza C, Hackethal S, Riccardi S, et al. Polysomnographic features of pregnancy: a systematic review. Sleep Med Rev 2020;50:101249.

13. Izci-Balserak B, Keenan BT, Corbitt C, et al. J Clin Sleep Med 2018;14(7):1161–8.

14.. Iczi-Balserak B, Lee K. Sleep and sleep disorders associated with pregnancy. In: Kryger M, Roth T, Dement W, editors. Principles and practice of sleep medicine. 6th edition. Philadelphia: Elsevier; 2017. p. 1525–39.

15. Pien GW, Fife D, Pack AI, et al. Changes in symptoms of sleep-disordered breathing during pregnancy. Sleep 2005;28(10):1299–305.

16. Bourjeily G, El Sabbagh R, Sawan P, et al. Epworth sleepiness scale scores and adverse pregnancy outcomes. Sleep Breath 2013;17(4): 1179–86.

17. Tsai SY, Lee PL, Lin JW, et al. Persistent and new-onset daytime sleepiness in pregnant women: a prospective observational cohort study. Int J Nurs Stud 2017;66:1–6.

18. Signal TL, Paine SJ, Sweeney B, et al. Prevalence of abnormal sleep duration and excessive daytime sleepiness in pregnancy and the role of sociodemographic factors: comparing pregnant women with women in the general population. Sleep Med 2014;15(12):1477–83.

19. Fernández-Alonso AM, Trabalón-Pastor M, Chedraui P, et al. Factors related to insomnia and sleepiness in the late third trimester of pregnancy. Arch Gynecol Obstet 2012;286(1):55–61.

20. Bourjeily G, Raker C, Chalhoub M, et al. Excessive daytime sleepiness in late pregnancy may not always be normal: results from a cross-sectional study. Sleep Breath 2013;17(2):735–40.

21. Bourjeily G, Danilack VA, Bublitz MH, et al. Obstructive sleep apnea in pregnancy is associated with adverse maternal outcomes: a national cohort. Sleep Med 2017;38:50–7.

22. Oyieng'o DO, Kirwa K, Tong I, et al. Restless legs symptoms and pregnancy and neonatal outcomes. Clin Ther 2016;38(2):256–64.

23. Robertson N, Flatley C, Kumar S. An Epworth Sleep Score ≥11 is associated with emergency operative birth and poor neonatal composite outcome at term. Aust N Z J Obstet Gynaecol 2020;60(1):49–54.

24. Tantrakul V, Numthavaj P, Guilleminault C, et al. Performance of screening questionnaires for obstructive sleep apnea during pregnancy: a systematic review and meta-analysis. Sleep Med Rev 2017; 36:96–106.

25. Tantrakul V, Sirijanchune P, Panburana P, et al. Screening of obstructive sleep apnea during pregnancy: differences in predictive values of questionnaires across trimesters. J Clin Sleep Med 2015; 11(2):157–63.

26. Picchietti DL, Hensley JG, Bainbridge JL, et al. Consensus clinical practice guidelines for the diagnosis and treatment of restless legs syndrome/willis-ekbom disease during pregnancy and lactation. Sleep Med Rev 2015;22:64–77.

27. Izci B, Riha RL, Martin SE, et al. The upper airway in pregnancy and pre-eclampsia. Am J Respir Crit Care Med 2003;167(2):137–40.

28. Sanapo L, Bublitz MH, Bourjeily G. Sleep disordered breathing, a novel, modifiable risk factor for hypertensive disorders of pregnancy. Curr Hypertens Rep 2020;22(4):28.

29. Loube DI, Poceta JS, Morales MC, et al. Self-reported snoring in pregnancy. Association with fetal outcome. Chest 1996;109(4):885–9.

30. Franklin KA, Holmgren PA, Jönsson F, et al. Snoring, pregnancy-induced hypertension, and growth retardation of the fetus. Chest 2000; 117(1):137–41.

31. Izci B, Vennelle M, Liston WA, et al. Sleep-disordered breathing and upper airway size in pregnancy and post-partum. Eur Respir J 2006;27(2): 321–7.

32. Edwards N, Blyton DM, Kirjavainen TT, et al. Hemodynamic responses to obstructive respiratory events during sleep are augmented in women with preeclampsia. Am J Hypertens 2001;14(11 Pt 1):1090–5.

33. Louis JM, Koch MA, Reddy UM, et al. Predictors of sleep-disordered breathing in pregnancy. Am J Obstet Gynecol 2018;218(5):521.e1–12.

34. Izci-Balserak B, Zhu B, Gurubhagavatula I, et al. A screening algorithm for obstructive sleep apnea in pregnancy. Ann Am Thorac Soc 2019;16(10): 1286–94.

35. Balserak BI, Zhu B, Grandner MA, et al. Obstructive sleep apnea in pregnancy: performance of a rapid screening tool. Sleep Breath 2019;23(2): 425–32.

36. Li L, Zhao K, Hua J, et al. Association between sleep-disordered breathing during pregnancy and maternal and fetal outcomes: an updated systematic review and meta-analysis. Front Neurol 2018;9:91.

37. Sedov ID, Anderson NJ, Dhillon AK, et al. Insomnia symptoms during pregnancy: a meta-analysis. J Sleep Res 2021;30(1):e13207.

38. Salari N, Darvishi N, Khaledi-Paveh B, et al. A systematic review and meta-analysis of prevalence of insomnia in the third trimester of pregnancy. BMC Pregnancy Childbirth 2021;21(1):284.

39. Lim KG, Morgenthaler TI, Katzka DA. Sleep and nocturnal gastroesophageal reflux: an update. Chest 2018;154(4):963–71.

40. Malfertheiner SF, Malfertheiner MV, Kropf S, et al. A prospective longitudinal cohort study: evolution of GERD symptoms during the course of pregnancy. BMC Gastroenterol 2012;12:131.

41. Reichner CA. Insomnia and sleep deficiency in pregnancy. Obstet Med 2015;8(4):168–71.

42. Howell MJ. Parasomnias: an updated review. Neurotherapeutics 2012;9(4):753–75.

43. Hedman C, Pohjasvaara T, Tolonen U, et al. Parasomnias decline during pregnancy. Acta Neurol Scand 2002;105(3):209–14.

44. Lara-Carrasco J, Simard V, Saint-Onge K, et al. Disturbed dreaming during the third trimester of pregnancy. Sleep Med 2014;15(6):694–700.

45.. DelRosso LM, Mogavero MP, Ferri R. Restless sleep disorder, restless legs syndrome, and periodic limb movement disorder-Sleep in motion! Pediatr Pulmonol 2021;1–8.

46. Bobrowski RA. Pulmonary physiology in pregnancy. Clin Obstet Gynecol 2010;53(2):285–300.

47. Kambam JR, Handte RE, Brown WU, et al. Effect of normal and preeclamptic pregnancies on the oxyhemoglobin dissociation curve. Anesthesiology 1986;65(4):426–7.

48. Shushan S, Sadan O, Lurie S, et al. Pregnancy-associated rhinitis. Am J Perinatol 2006;23(7): 431–3.

49. Lee J, Eklund EE, Lambert-Messerlian G, et al. Serum progesterone levels in pregnant women with obstructive sleep apnea: a case control study. J Womens Health (Larchmt) 2017;26(3):259–65.

50. Lui B, Burey L, Ma X, et al. Obstructive sleep apnea is associated with adverse maternal outcomes using a United States multistate database cohort, 2007-2014. Int J Obstet Anesth 2021;45:74–82.

51. Facco FL, Ouyang DW, Zee PC, et al. Sleep disordered breathing in a high-risk cohort prevalence and severity across pregnancy. Am J Perinatol 2014;31(10):899–904.

52. Liu L, Su G, Wang S, et al. The prevalence of obstructive sleep apnea and its association with pregnancy-related health outcomes: a systematic review and meta-analysis. Sleep Breath 2019; 23(2):399–412.

53. Bourjeily G, Raker C, Paglia MJ, et al. Patient and provider perceptions of sleep disordered breathing assessment during prenatal care: a survey-based observational study. Ther Adv Respir Dis 2012; 6(4):211–9.

54. Facco FL, Ouyang DW, Zee PC, et al. Development of a pregnancy-specific screening tool for sleep apnea. J Clin Sleep Med 2012;8(4):389–94.

55. Pearson F, Batterham AM, Cope S. The STOP-bang questionnaire as a screening tool for obstructive sleep apnea in pregnancy. J Clin Sleep Med 2019;15(5):705–10.

56. Siriyotha S, Tantrakul V, Plitphonganphim S, et al. Prediction models of obstructive sleep apnea in pregnancy: a systematic review and meta-analysis of model performance. Diagnostics (Basel) 2021;11(6):1097.

57. Dominguez JE, Grotegut CA, Cooter M, et al. Screening extremely obese pregnant women for obstructive sleep apnea. Am J Obstet Gynecol 2018;219(6):613.e1–10.

58. Facco FL, Lopata V, Wolsk JM, et al. Can we use home sleep testing for the evaluation of sleep apnea in obese pregnant women? Sleep Disord 2019;2019:3827579.

59. O'Brien LM, Bullough AS, Shelgikar AV, et al. Validation of Watch-PAT-200 against polysomnography during pregnancy. J Clin Sleep Med 2012;8(3): 287–94.

60. Bourjeily G, Fung JY, Sharkey KM, et al. Airflow limitations in pregnant women suspected of sleep-disordered breathing. Sleep Med 2014;15(5):550–5.

61. Reid J, Glew RA, Mink J, et al. Hemodynamic response to upper airway obstruction in

hypertensive and normotensive pregnant women. Can Respir J 2016,2016:0816494,

62. Link BN, Eid C, Bublitz MH, et al. Pulse transit time in pregnancy: a new way to diagnose and classify sleep disordered breathing? Sleep 2019;42(5): zsz022.

63. Yinon D, Lowenstein L, Suraya S, et al. Pre-eclampsia is associated with sleep-disordered breathing and endothelial dysfunction. Eur Respir J 2006;27(2):328–33.

64. Somers VK, Dyken ME, Clary MP, et al. Sympathetic neural mechanisms in obstructive sleep apnea. J Clin Invest 1995;96(4):1897–904.

65. Ravishankar S, Bourjeily G, Lambert-Messerlian G, et al. Evidence of placental hypoxia in maternal sleep disordered breathing. Pediatr Dev Pathol 2015;18(5):380–6.

66. Kidron D, Bar-Lev Y, Tsarfaty I, et al. The effect of maternal obstructive sleep apnea on the placenta. Sleep 2019;42(6):zsz072.

67. Guilleminault C, Kreutzer M, Chang JL. Pregnancy, sleep disordered breathing and treatment with nasal continuous positive airway pressure. Sleep Med 2004;5(1):43–51.

68. Edwards N, Blyton DM, Kirjavainen T, et al. Nasal continuous positive airway pressure reduces sleep-induced blood pressure increments in pre-eclampsia. Am J Respir Crit Care Med 2000; 162(1):252–7.

69. Chen SJ, Shi L, Bao YP, et al. Prevalence of restless legs syndrome during pregnancy: a systematic review and meta-analysis. Sleep Med Rev 2018;40: 43–54.

70. Panvatvanich S, Lolekha P. Restless legs syndrome in pregnant Thai women: prevalence, predictive factors, and natural course. J Clin Neurol 2019; 15(1):97–101.

71. Godau J, Klose U, Di Santo A, et al. Multiregional brain iron deficiency in restless legs syndrome. Mov Disord 2008;23(8):1184–7.

72. Earley CJ, Barker PB, Horská A, et al. MRI-determined regional brain iron concentrations in early- and late-onset restless legs syndrome. Sleep Med 2006;7(5):458–61.

73. Chen PH, Liou KC, Chen CP, et al. Risk factors and prevalence rate of restless legs syndrome among pregnant women in Taiwan. Sleep Med 2012; 13(9):1153–7.

74. Shang X, Yang J, Guo Y, et al. Restless legs syndrome among pregnant women in China: prevalence and risk factors. Sleep Breath 2015;19(3):1093–9.

75. Hübner A, Krafft A, Gadient S, et al. Characteristics and determinants of restless legs syndrome in pregnancy: a prospective study. Neurology 2013; 80(8):738–42.

76. Vahdat M, Sariri E, Miri S, et al. Prevalence and associated features of restless legs syndrome in a population of Iranian women during pregnancy. Int J Gynaecol Obstet 2013;123(1):46–9.

77. Gupta R, Dhyani M, Kendzerska T, et al. Restless legs syndrome and pregnancy: provalence, possible pathophysiological mechanisms and treatment. Acta Neurol Scand 2016;133(5):320–9.

78. Garbazza C, Manconi M. Management strategies for restless legs syndrome/willis-ekbom disease during pregnancy. Sleep Med Clin 2018;13(3): 335–48.

79. Goodman JD, Brodie C, Ayida GA. Restless leg syndrome in pregnancy. BMJ 1988;297(6656): 1101–2.

80. Manconi M, Govoni V, De Vito A, et al. Restless legs syndrome and pregnancy. Neurology 2004;63(6): 1065–9.

81. Cesnik E, Casetta I, Turri M, et al. Transient RLS during pregnancy is a risk factor for the chronic idiopathic form. Neurology 2010;75(23):2117–20.

82. Allen RP, Picchietti DL, Garcia-Borreguero D, et al. Restless legs syndrome/willis-ekbom disease diagnostic criteria: updated International Restless Legs Syndrome Study Group (IRLSSG) consensus criteria–history, rationale, description, and significance. Sleep Med 2014;15(8):860–73.

83. Garcia-Borreguero D, Kohnen R, Silber MH, et al. The long-term treatment of restless legs syndrome/Willis-Ekbom disease: evidence-based guidelines and clinical consensus best practice guidance: a report from the International Restless Legs Syndrome Study Group. Sleep Med 2013; 14(7):675–84.

84. Garcia-Borreguero D, Silber MH, Winkelman JW, et al. Guidelines for the first-line treatment of restless legs syndrome/willis-ekbom disease, prevention and treatment of dopaminergic augmentation: a combined task force of the IRLSSG, EURLSSG, and the RLS-foundation. Sleep Med 2016;21:1–11.

85. Sharon D, Allen RP, Martinez-Martin P, et al. Validation of the self-administered version of the international Restless Legs Syndrome study group severity rating scale - the sIRLS. Sleep Med 2019;54:94–100.

86. Dostal M, Weber-Schoendorfer C, Sobesky J, et al. Pregnancy outcome following use of levodopa, pramipexol e, ropinirole, and rotigotine for restless legs syndrome during pregnancy: a case series. Eur J Neurol 2013;20(9):1241–6.

87. Eroglu C, Allen NJ, Susman MW, et al. Gabapentin receptor alpha2delta-1 is a neuronal thrombospondin receptor responsible for excitatory CNS synaptogenesis. Cell 2009;139(2):380–92.

88. Ohman I, Vitols S, Tomson T. Pharmacokinetics of gabapentin during delivery, in the neonatal period, and lactation: does a fetal accumulation occur during pregnancy? Epilepsia 2005;46(10):1621–4.

89. Briggs GGFR, Yaffe SJ. Drugs in pregnancy and lactation. 10th edition. Philadelphia (PA): Lippincott Williams & Wilkins; 2015.

90. Kargas GA, Kargas SA, Bruyere HJ Jr, et al. Perinatal mortality due to interaction of diphenhydramine and temazepam. N Engl J Med 1985; 313(22):1417–8.

91. Wen X, Belviso N, Murray E, et al. Association of gestational opioid exposure and risk of major and minor congenital malformations. JAMA Netw Open 2021;4(4):e215708.

92. Bateman BT, Hernandez-Diaz S, Straub L, et al. Association of first trimester prescription opioid use with congenital malformations in the offspring: population based cohort study. BMJ 2021;372:n102.

93. Javaheri S, Barbe F, Campos-Rodriguez F, et al. Sleep apnea: types, mechanisms, and clinical cardiovascular consequences. J Am Coll Cardiol 2017;69(7):841–58.

94. Lanfrachi PA, Pepin JL, Somers VK. Cardiovascular physiology: autonomic control in health and in sleep disorders. In: Kryger M, Roth T, Dement W, editors. Principles and practice of sleep medicine. 6th edition. Philadelphia: Elsevier; 2017. p. 142–54.

95. O'Connor GT, Caffo B, Newman AB, et al. Prospective study of sleep-disordered breathing and hypertension: the sleep heart health study. Am J Respir Crit Care Med 2009;179(12):1159–64.

96. Seravalle G, Mancia G, Grassi G. Sympathetic nervous system, sleep, and hypertension. Curr Hypertens Rep 2018;20(9):74.

97. Leproult R, Van Cauter E. Role of sleep and sleep loss in hormonal release and metabolism. Endocr Dev 2010;17:11–21.

98. Tiwari R, Tam DNH, Shah J, et al. Effects of sleep intervention on glucose control: a narrative review of clinical evidence. Prim Care Diabetes 2021; 15(4):635–41.

99. Wangel AM, Molin J, Ostman M, et al. Emergency cesarean sections can be predicted by markers for stress, worry and sleep disturbances in first-time mothers. Acta Obstet Gynecol Scand 2011; 90(3):238–44.

100. Serón-Ferré M, Ducsay CA, Valenzuela GJ. Circadian rhythms during pregnancy. Endocr Rev 1993;14(5):594–609.

101. Khalyfa A, Mutskov V, Carreras A, et al. Sleep fragmentation during late gestation induces metabolic perturbations and epigenetic changes in adiponectin gene expression in male adult offspring mice. Diabetes 2014;63(10):3230–41.

102. Chang JJ, Pien GW, Duntley SP, et al. Sleep deprivation during pregnancy and maternal and fetal outcomes: is there a relationship? Sleep Med Rev 2010;14(2):107–14.

103. Micheli K, Komninos I, Bagkeris E, et al. Sleep patterns in late pregnancy and risk of preterm birth and fetal growth restriction. Epidemiology 2011; 22(5):738–44.

104. Bonzini M, Palmer KT, Coggon D, et al. Shift work and pregnancy outcomes: a systematic review with meta-analysis of currently available epidemiological studies. BJOG 2011;118(12):1429–37.

105. Warland J, Dorrian J, Morrison JL, et al. Maternal sleep during pregnancy and poor fetal outcomes: a scoping review of the literature with meta-analysis. Sleep Med Rev 2018;41:197–219.

106. Brown NT, Turner JM, Kumar S. The intrapartum and perinatal risks of sleep-disordered breathing in pregnancy: a systematic review and metaanalysis. Am J Obstet Gynecol 2018;219(2):147–61.e1.

107. Dadi AF, Miller ER, Bisetegn TA, et al. Global burden of antenatal depression and its association with adverse birth outcomes: an umbrella review. BMC Public Health 2020;20(1):173.

108. Wichniak A, Wierzbicka A, Jernajczyk W. Sleep as a biomarker for depression. Int Rev Psychiatry 2013;25(5):632–45.

109. Dørheim SK, Bjorvatn B, Eberhard-Gran M. Insomnia and depressive symptoms in late pregnancy: a population-based study. Behav Sleep Med 2012;10(3):152–66.

Evaluation and Management of Snoring

Yoke-Yeow Yap, MD, MMed (ORL-HNS)

KEYWORDS

- Snoring • Sleep-disordered breathing • Obstructive sleep apnea • Phenotypes
- Nasal airway complex • Mouth breathing

KEY POINTS

- Snoring can be harmless (primary) or a symptom of sleep-disordered breathing (SDB) (secondary) and should alert the physician to evaluate the patient for risks thereof.
- Phenotypes of snoring and SDB are anatomic and nonanatomic and identifying these phenotypes and their interrelationships are critical to effective therapy.
- Mouth breathing alerts the physician to nasal airway obstruction, signals orofacial growth changes in children, and heralds the progression of SDB.
- Systematic evaluation to establish phenotypes includes assessing sleep habits, comorbidities, upper airway examination, polysomnography, and drug-induced sleep endoscopy.
- Strategies for treatment should be personalized and precise to the phenotype(s) to achieve the most benefit.

INTRODUCTION

Snoring is biomechanically a vibratory noise produced in sleep from a cyclical obstruction and reopening of the upper airway at approximately 50x/s[1], arising from the soft palate (100%), pharynx (53.8%), lateral pharyngeal wall (42.3%), epiglottis (42.3%), and tongue base (26.9%).[2] Solitary palatal fluttering is seen in simple snorers, palate & lateral pharyngeal wall vibration in mild-to-moderate obstructive sleep apnea (OSA), and combined palate-lateral pharyngeal wall-tongue base-epiglottis vibration in severe OSA.[2] Snoring in OSA occurs mostly in apnea-terminating hyperpneas when turbulence is maximum.[3]

SNORING AND SLEEP-DISORDERED BREATHING

Snoring indicates a 5x increased risk of OSA.[4] In an online survey of 664 women and 575 men in the United Kingdom aged 18 to 100 years, snoring was reported in 38% of men and 30.4% of women, while pauses in breathing was reported in 8.7% of men and 5.6% of women.[5] In women, regular snoring is associated with increased risk of coronary heart disease (risk ratio (RR): 2.18) and stroke (RR 1.88)[6]. Primary snoring is not associated with sleepiness or medical hazards, whereas secondary snoring is symptomatic of sleep-disordered breathing (SDB)—a spectrum from upper airway resistance syndrome (UARS), to mild, moderate, and severe OSA. Population-based studies show 9% to 38% of adults more than 18 years old have OSA—13% to 33% in men and 6% to 19% in women and increases to 90% in men and 78% in women greater than 65 years of age.[7] Multiple systemic chronic illnesses are associated with SDB.[8] Polysomnographic classification, however, does not correlate well with the quality of life and comorbidities of SDB, nor does it guide treatment or predict outcome in a widely heterogenous problem.

CAUSES AND PHENOTYPES OF SNORING AND SLEEP-DISORDERED BREATHING

Phenotyping and integrated analysis of multiple factors, augmented by machine learning, is needed to arrive at unique and meaningful categories to

KPJ Johor Specialist Hospital, 39b Jalan Abdul Samad, Johor Bahru 80100, Malaysia
E-mail address: yokeyeow@gmail.com

Sleep Med Clin 17 (2022) 25–39
https://doi.org/10.1016/j.jsmc.2021.10.010
1556-407X/22/© 2021 Elsevier Inc. All rights reserved.

sleep.theclinics.com

prognosticate and guide decision-making in the future treatment of SDB (**Fig. 1**).[9]

Broad phenotyping includes anatomic and nonanatomic factors (**Fig. 2**) but patients do not always fit neatly into these categories (**Box 1**). Multiple factors are usually present, and their dynamic interrelationship needs to be adequately appreciated in strategizing timing and type(s) of therapy[11] (**Fig. 3**.)

Anatomic Factors

The upper airway consists of a skeletal "container" with soft tissue "contents" of the nasal airway complex (NAC) and the pharynx (**Table 1**). Cephalometric analysis in patients with OSA show increased lower anterior facial height and vertical growth pattern (long and narrow faces), an inferior position of hyoid bone, decreased pharyngeal airway space, decreased length of the cranial base and cranial base angle, relatively smaller maxilla and mandible, retro-positioned mandibles, and also increased length, thickness, and surface area of soft palate.[12] Decreased lower anterior facial height is predictive of severe OSA.[13] Retrognathia is much more common in severe OSA than in snorers.[14] Clockwise rotation and shorter mandibles are also associated with OSA.[12]

The NAC contributes more than 50% of airway resistance with the area of greatest resistance at the internal and external nasal valves.[15] Nasal obstruction worsens the respiratory disturbance index (RDI),[16] OSA severity,[17] and impairs sleep quality in allergic and nonallergic rhinitis.[18,19] An acute maxillary angle, narrow maxillary width, and high arched palate are skeletal characteristics associated with persistent nasal obstruction contributing to SDB.[20] 85% of patients with OSA with nasal obstruction has septal deviation and/or turbinate hypertrophy.[14] Inferior turbinate hypertrophy is found in 93% to 97% of snorers and OSA.[21]

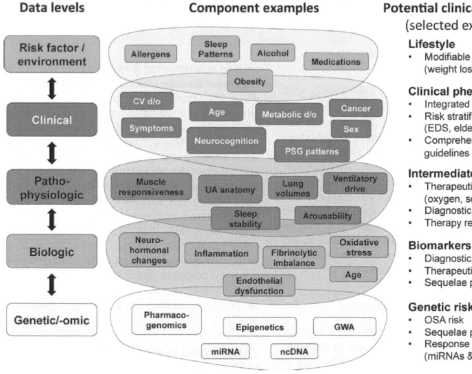

Fig. 1. Data levels in obstructive sleep apnea (OSA) phenotyping and the potential benefits.[9] Illustration of phenotyping data levels (risk factor/environment, clinical, pathophysiologic, biological, gen-etic/omic) in OSA and the potential benefits (right-hand column). Each level shows only some examples of the potential components (not intended to be comprehensive). Arrows signify integration of the levels to better understand their relationship in OSA. CCC, complete concentric palatal collapse, CV d/o, cardiovascular disorders, EDS, excessive daytime sleepiness, GWA, genome-wide associations, HTN, hypertension, IL, interleukin, miRNA, microRNA, ncDNA, non-coding DNA, PALM, Passive Pcrit, Arousal threshold, Loop gain, and upper airway Muscle responsiveness model, PSG, polysomnographic, UA, upper airway. Taken from Zinchuk AV, Gentry MJ, Concato J, Yaggi HK. Phenotypes in obstructive sleep apnea: A definition, examples and evolution of approaches. Sleep Med Rev. 2017;35:113-123. doi:10.1016/j.smrv.2016.10.002.

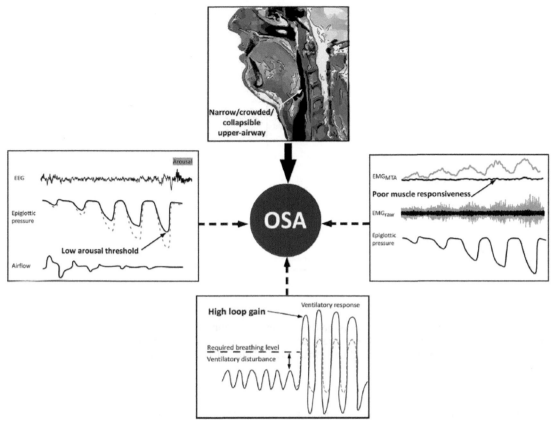

Fig. 2. Schematic of the anatomic and nonanatomical causes of OSA.[10]. Taken from Carberry JC, Amatoury J, Eckert DJ. Personalized Management Approach for OSA. Chest. 2018;153(3):744-755. doi:10.1016/j.chest.2017.06.011.

The pharynx of patients with OSA is narrower,[22] rounder (smaller transverse diameter) versus oval (larger transverse diameter),[23] more collapsible and must expand more to facilitate airflow. Macroglossia,[24] adenotonsillar hypertrophy,[25] thickening of the lateral pharyngeal walls (attributed to obesity, inflammation, or vascular volume) crowd the airway further. The presence of tongue scalloping is strongly predictive of abnormal AHI and nocturnal hypoxia[26,27] caused by a large tongue, small mandible, or high-arched palate. A short lingual frenulum at birth also leads to OSA[28] and sleep disturbance (odds ratio (OR): 2.98).[29] It is associated with 5x increased risk of OSA in children aged 3 to 17 (n = 135),[30] due to narrowing of the maxillary arch and elongation of the soft palate,[31] which is a result of loss of tongue-palate coupling necessary for maxillary growth.

Dynamic Factors

End-expiratory collapse occurs when constricting forces (ie, endoluminal negative inspiratory pressure and extraluminal parapharyngeal fat volume) overwhelm the expanding force of pharyngeal dilators.[32] This imbalance increases the critical closing pressure (Pcrit)—a more positive (or less negative) Pcrit indicates a more collapsible airway. Pcrit is increased by a larger neck circumference, soft palate length, and hyomental distance.[33] Reduced end-expiratory lung volume (EELV) in the obese also increases Pcrit and aggravates OSA.[34]

Pharyngeal dilator function. Altered neuromuscular function and reflexes of pharyngeal dilators are seen in OSA—the genioglossus demonstrates lower tonic activity[35] and increased phasic activation in response to apnea.[36] Neuromuscular responses—to hypoxia, reduced airway diameter,

---

Box 1
Anatomic and non-anatomic subtypes of SDB[10]

- Upper airway obstruction
- Pharyngeal dilator function
- Increased loop gain
- Low arousal threshold

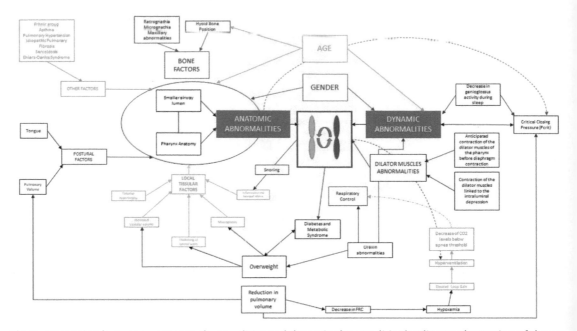

Fig. 3. Interaction between anatomic abnormalities and dynamic abnormalities leading to obstruction of the upper respiratory tract. (*Adapted from* Deflandre E, Gerdom A, Lamarque C, Bertrand B. Understanding Pathophysiological Concepts Leading to Obstructive Apnea. *Obes Surg.* 2018;28(8):2560-2571. https://doi.org/10.1007/s11695-018-3325-6)[11]

and airway pressure—fatigues by as much as 50%[37] in OSA and protective reflexes are impaired as well.[38]

High loop gain (LG) is an exaggerated ventilatory response to CO_2 changes and a third of patients with OSA have high LG whereby a >5 L/min increase in minute volume (MV) is seen in response to a 1 L/min reduction in MV. This creates a hypoventilation–hyperventilation cycle, respiratory instability, and increased apneas.[39]

Arousal threshold may be reduced in patients with OSA whereby sudden arousals augment pharyngeal dilator muscle activity to reopen the airway. The hyperventilatory response drives down CO_2 below the chemical apnea threshold resulting in central apneas. Hypocapnia also impairs the dilator function by decreasing the neural output.[40] A low arousal threshold (ArTH > −15 cm H2O) can be predicted by a clinical score whereby:

(AHI >30)+(nadir SaO2 >82.5%)+($F_{hypopneas}$ > 58.3%) ≥2 predicts low ArTH in 84% (sens 80%, spec 88%)[41]

"Mouth Breathing Syndrome"

Mouth breathing is a red flag for SDB—alerting us to the presence of nasal obstruction from allergic rhinitis (81.4%), enlarged adenoids (79.2%), enlarged tonsils (12.6%), and deviation of the nasal septum (1.0%)[42] (**Fig. 4.**) In children, this heralds the perilous progression of SDB. Airway resistance (+7.2 cmH2O x L^{-1} x s^{-1}), AHI (+41/h), and obstructive apnea-hypopneas are increased in oral breathing versus nasal breathing during sleep.[43] This is explained by the reduced pharyngeal diameter, pharyngeal dilator shortening, and impaired dilator function in mouth breathing.[44,45]

Mouth breathing was reported in 17% of the population of Nagahama City, Japan (n = 9804). Worsening of asthma by 85% was found in those with mouth breathing alone, by 2.2x in those with allergic rhinitis alone and 4x when mouth breathing, and allergic rhinitis coexisted.[46] A systematic review

Table 1
Anatomic framework for SDB

	Skeletal (Container)	Soft Tissue (Content)
Nasal Airway Complex	Maxilla Pyriform aperture Hard palate	Turbinates Septum Alar valve
Pharyngeal Airway	Maxilla Mandible Epiglottis Hyoid	Adenoids Tonsils Tongue & tongue-tie Tongue base

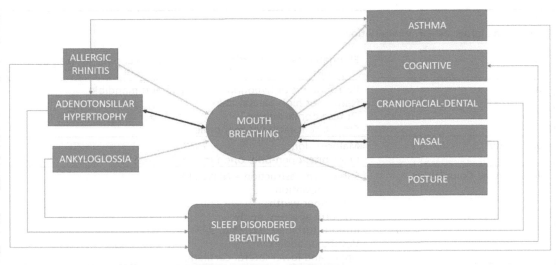

Fig. 4. Causes and consequences of the mouth breathing syndrome.

mouth breathers in Brazil showed increased malocclusion, with Angle Class II, division 1 (33%) greater than Class I (7%).[47] Postural changes such as forward head position, higher head projection, and shoulder asymmetry are also seen in mouth breathers.[48]

EVALUATION OF THE SNORING PATIENT

The aims of evaluation are to identify the phenotypic patterns and their interrelationships (as outlined above), grade severity of disorder, establish the baseline for intervention, and guide treatment options. A systematic evaluation should proceed as follows:

Sleep health history

Snoring habit
Timeline, periodicity in the night, association with drugs or alcohol, association with body position, gasping, choking, and witnessed apneas.

Underlying airway disorders
Rhinitis, tonsillitis, respiratory disorders.

Sleep quality
Insomnia, nocturnal awakenings, daytime sleepiness, inattention, reduction in work or school performance.

SDB symptoms in children[49,50]
Hyperactive behavior, bed-wetting, night terrors, bruxism, inattention, sleepiness, poor school performance, stertor, dry mouth, or observed mouth breathing.

SDB symptoms in adults
Early morning headaches, loss of libido, mood changes, erectile dysfunction, nocturia.

Comorbidities

Hypertension
Increased risk of systemic hypertension by 37% with AHI ≥ 30[51] and 24% in a twofold increase in Rapid Eye Movement Apnea-Hypopnea Index (REM AHI).[52]

Cardiovascular
Relative odds of heart failure are 2.38, stroke 1.58, and coronary heart disease 1.27 comparing highest-quartile versus lowest quartile AHI.[53]

Diabetes mellitus
Hazard ratios of developing diabetes for mild, moderate, and severe OSA are 0.94, 1.28, and 1.71 compared with non-OSA population.[54]

Cognitive decline
Meta-analysis of cohort studies (n = 19,940) showed increased cognitive impairment or dementia (RR = 1.69) in individuals with SDB.[55]

Systemic examination

BMI/obesity
Severe obesity is associated with moderate-to-severe sleep apnea in 65% of males and 23% of females.[56] Neck circumference correlates well with increased soft tissue volume of the tongue and lateral pharyngeal walls[57]

a. Cranial dysmorphisms
b. Hypothyroidism or acromegaly

Upper airway examination

(**Table 2**). Sites and patterns of obstruction (ie, skeletal and/or soft tissue, overcrowded or collapsing, static or dynamic) should be identified by flexible endoscopic examination.

Table 2
Systematic upper airway examination

Face	Elongated face, underdeveloped lower face, poor lip seal, open mouth
Jaws	Retrognathic or hypognathic maxilla and mandible Narrow or high palatal arch Obtuse gonial angles Clockwise rotation of mandible
Oral cavity	Malocclusion Cross-bite, open-bite, open mouth
Nasal Airway Complex	Subjective obstruction – NOSE(20) scale[58] Septal deviation Nasal floor width Pyriform aperture angle Inferior turbinate size (**Fig. 5**)[59] Vestibular bodies[60] Upper and lower lateral cartilages
Nasopharynx	Adenoid size
Soft palate	Bulk Length Angle – oblique, intermediate, vertical[61] (**Fig. 6**) Shape of upper pharynx[62]
Tongue	Size Scalloping Anterior and posterior tongue-tie Tongue range of motion (**Fig. 7**)[63] Friedman tongue position (or modified mallampati score)
Tongue base and epiglottis	Size of tongue base Size of lingual tonsils Shape of lower pharynx – type A, B, C (see **Fig. 6**)[61]
Lateral pharyngeal wall	Size of tonsils Narrowing of lateral walls.
Posture	Forward head position, shoulder asymmetry, lumbar lordosis

Polysomnography

This remains the gold standard for differentiating primary snorers from SDB and assessing their severity. A level I, fully attended sleep study provides complete information but may be inaccessible to most and is difficult and costly to administer. Levels II and III studies are cheaper and more comfortable but offer limited information. Level IV studies are useful only as a screening tool. Type of study should be selected based on possible comorbidities, sleep disorders, and the information and accuracy provided by the modality (**Table 3**). With less information, more clinical assessment is needed, and one should be ready to upgrade to a level I study when in doubt.

Imaging

a. Lateral cephalogram[64] (**Fig. 8**)
b. Magnetic resonance imaging (MRI)/computerized tomography (CT) scan could assess nasal airway complex, pharyngeal airway; soft tissue bulk of tongue, tongue base, and parapharyngeal space.

Drug-induced sleep endoscopy (DISE)

DISE identifies the site(s) and severity of the upper airway. The most accepted convention is the VOTE classification by Kerizian, and colleagues[65] (**Fig. 9**). A review of 1249 patients with OSA undergoing DISE showed palatal (81%) and tongue base (46.6%) collapse to be the most prevalent (**Fig. 10**) while 68.1% were multilevel.[66]

MANAGEMENT OF SNORING & OSA

Treatments for snoring and OSA include a variety of non-pharmacologic, pharmacologic and surgical options. Selection of therapy and their timing should be based on:

1 Age – child or adult, prepubertal or postpubertal.

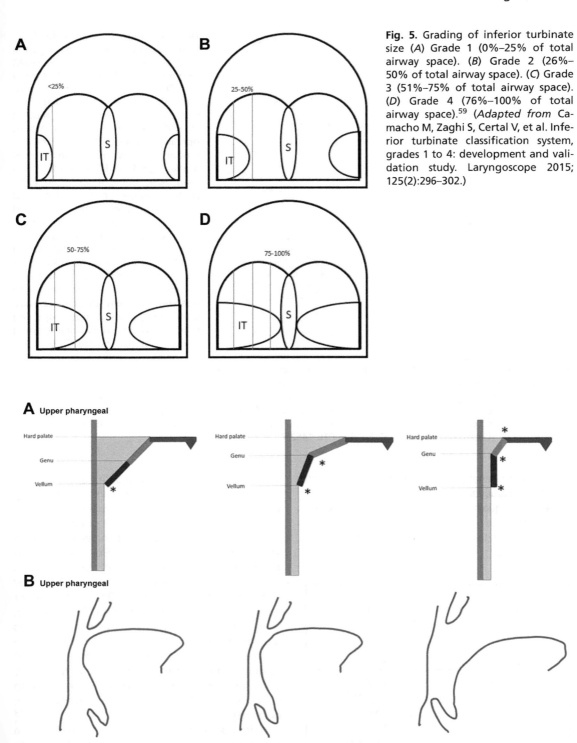

Fig. 5. Grading of inferior turbinate size (*A*) Grade 1 (0%–25% of total airway space). (*B*) Grade 2 (26%–50% of total airway space). (*C*) Grade 3 (51%–75% of total airway space). (*D*) Grade 4 (76%–100% of total airway space).[59] (*Adapted from* Camacho M, Zaghi S, Certal V, et al. Inferior turbinate classification system, grades 1 to 4: development and validation study. Laryngoscope 2015; 125(2):296–302.)

Fig. 6. Patterns of upper pharyngeal (*A*) and lower pharyngeal (*B*) vertical shape are depicted. Narrowing (*) occurs in the upper pharynx at the following locations: oblique pattern at the velum; intermediate at the velum and genu; and vertical at velum, genu, and hard palate. For the lower pharynx, a modified Moore Classification of the lower pharynx is shown (*B*). Airway types include proximal (type A), proximal and distal obstruction (type B), and obstruction at the retroepiglottic/vallecular tongue segment (type C). (*Adapted from* Woodson BT. A method to describe the pharyngeal airway. Laryngoscope. 2015;125(5):1233-1238. https://doi.org/10.1002/lary.24972)[61.]

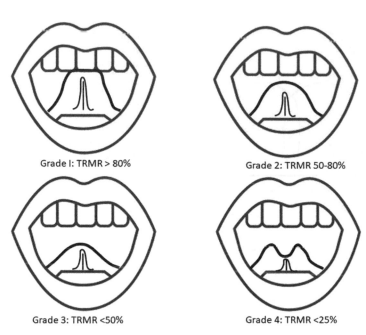

Grade I: TRMR > 80%

Grade 2: TRMR 50-80%

Grade 3: TRMR <50%

Grade 4: TRMR <25%

Fig. 7. A grading scale for the functional classification of ankyloglossia is proposed based on the TRMR [tongue range of motion ratio] (ratio of MOTTIP [interincisal mouth opening with tongue tip to maxillary incisive papillae at the roof of mouth] to MIO[maximal interincisal mouth opening]). Grade 1: tongue range of motion ratio is greater than 80%, grade 2 50% to 80%, grade 3 less than 50%, grade 4 less than 25%. Higher grades reflect decreased tongue mobility and increased severity of tongue-tie. The illustrations here demonstrate the deficit in the mobility of the tongue tip relative to MIO. With increasing ankyloglossia, the tongue tip is unable to touch the incisive papilla unless the mouth opening is closed to some extent. Considering grade 3, mouth opening is limited to 50% of maximal opening in order for the tongue tip to reach the incisive papilla. For grade 4, mouth opening is limited to 25% of MIO for the tongue tip to reach the incisive papilla[63]. Yoon A, Zaghi S, Weitzman R, et al. Toward a functional definition of ankyloglossia: validating current grading scales for lingual frenulum length and tongue mobility in 1052 subjects. Sleep Breath. 2017;21(3):767-775. doi:10.1007/s11325-016-1452-7. Adapted from Yoon A, Zaghi S, Weitzman R, et al. Toward a functional definition of ankyloglossia: validating current grading scales for lingual frenulum length and tongue mobility in 1052 subjects. Sleep Breath. 2017;21(3):767-775. doi:10.1007/s11325-016-1452-7.

2 Phenotype – anatomic or functional, skeletal or soft tissue obstruction, static or dynamic obstruction.

3 Severity – quality of life, polysomnographic data, comorbidities.

4 Risk for anesthesia and/or type of surgery being considered.

Table 3
Choice of sleep study based on the type of sleep disorder and information needed

Types of Sleep Disorder	Information Needed
Psychological	EEG, EMG (level I or II)
Movement Disorders	EEG, EMG (level I or II)
Sleep-Breathing Disorders	Airflow, effort, oximetry (level III)
Positional OSA	+ Actigraphy (level I or II)
UARS	+ EEG (level I or II)
REM OSA	+ EEG (level I or II)
Central Sleep Apnea	* Airflow
Cheyne-Stokes Respiration	* Airflow

Patients often require trials of therapy and combinations of different modalities in phases, taking into account the efficacies, invasiveness, cost-risk-benefit analyses, and patient preferences.

General measures. General measures include weight loss and sleep hygiene. Posture modifications may help in position-related OSA.

Positive airway pressure therapy. PAP therapy includes continuous PAP and Bilevel PAP, either manually or automatically titrated. PAP therapy, while not reversing primary causes of SDB, is effective for all severities of OSA, eliminating snoring and normalizing AHI in 90% of cases.[67] Urgent cases of moderate-to-severe OSA with multiple comorbidities and high surgical risk benefit from early therapy. PAP lowers blood pressure in a dose-dependent way,[68] improves cognition[69] and improves cardiovascular outcomes in the long term.[66] PAP compliance is a challenge with nonadherence rate remaining at 34% in a 20-year review.[70]

Myofunctional therapy. Myofunctional therapy (MFT) aims to restore nasal breathing, upper airway reflexes, lip closure and tone, tongue posture and tone, mandible position, and orofacial growth. Exercises target pharyngeal dilators, elevators and tensors of the soft palate,

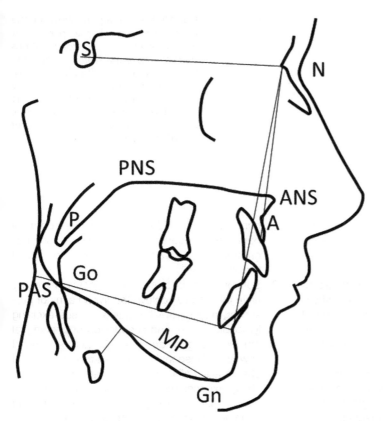

Fig. 8. Cephalometric figure. (*Adapted from* Riley RW, Powell NB, Guilleminault C. Inferior mandibular osteotomy and hyoid myotomy suspension for obstructive sleep apnea: a review of 55 patients. J Oral Maxillofac Surg 1989;47(2):160)

and lateral pharyngeal wall muscles. MFT has been shown to reduce AHI by 50% in adults and 62% in children along with improvements in oxygen saturation, sleepiness, and snoring.[71] It corrects mouth breathing in children alongside nasal interventions and prevents adult OSA.[72] It is also useful in improving CPAP compliance.[73] Standardized regimes for comparison are needed moving forward.

Medical and Surgical Therapy for Nasal Obstruction

Nasal airway optimization is a prerequisite to CPAP or surgery. It is also critical in the management of childhood SDB and mouth breathing.

Twelve weeks of intranasal corticosteroid therapy in OSA with AR significantly improves sleep quality, lowest oxygen saturation, and AHI.[74,75] Surgery for nasal obstruction includes turbinate reduction, alar valve repair, septoplasty, and endoscopic sinus surgery. A systematic review (n = 158) showed isolated nasal surgery conducted for OSA reduces AHI (by 4.15) and ESS.[76] Nasal surgery reduces average therapeutic CPAP pressures from 11.6 ± 2.2 cm H_2O to 9.5 ± 2.0 cm H_2O and increases adherence.[77,78]

Drug therapies for loop gain and arousal threshold

O_2 therapy reduces LG and OSA severity, as does carbonic anhydrase inhibitors such as

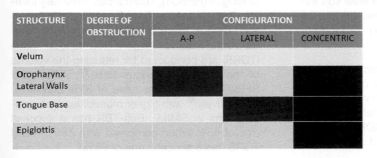

STRUCTURE	DEGREE OF OBSTRUCTION	CONFIGURATION		
		A-P	LATERAL	CONCENTRIC
Velum				
Oropharynx Lateral Walls				
Tongue Base				
Epiglottis				

Fig. 9. The VOTE classification for DISE. (*Adapted from* Kezirian EJ, Hohenhorst W, de Vries N. Drug-induced sleep endoscopy: the VOTE classification. Eur Arch Otorhinolaryngol. 2011;268(8):1233-1236. (https://doi.org/10.1007/s00405-011-1633-865)

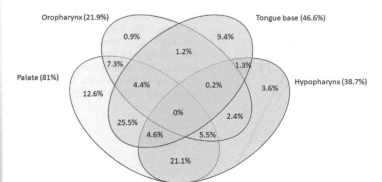

Fig. 10. Venn diagram showing the prevalence of collapse per upper airway level and the combinations thereof. (*Adapted from* Vroegop AV, Vanderveken OM, Boudewyns AN, et al. Drug-induced sleep endoscopy in sleep-disordered breathing: report on 1,249 cases. Laryngoscope. 2014;124(3):797-802. https://doi.org/10.1002/lary.24479.)[66]

acetazolamide which reduces OSA severity and LG by 40%. Zonisamide reduces OSA severity, and stabilization of CO_2 and hypercapnia can prevent hypoventilation and unstable respiratory control. Combining O_2 therapy with a hypnotic to reduce LG and increase the arousal threshold yields major reductions in OSA severity.[39] Arousal threshold is increased by 28% and 48%, with eszopiclone and trazodone, concomitantly reducing the AHI.[41]

Upper airway stimulation. Upper airway stimulation with a hypoglossal nerve implant normalizes ESS scores by 78% and achieves greater than 50% reduction of AHI in 75% of patients (n = 71) in a 5-year outcome review of patients who failed CPAP[79]

Oral appliances. Oral appliances for OSA include mandibular advancement devices (MAD) (as 1-piece monoblocks or 2-piece biblocks), or tongue-stabilizing devices (TSD).[80] Patients prefer MADs than TSDs despite similar efficacy in reducing AHI.[81] Mean AHI can be reduced by 13.6/h in a meta-nalytic review of RCTs involving oral appliances.[82] Compared with CPAP, MAD compliance is better by 1.1 h/night, explaining the similar health outcomes despite greater efficacy in CPAP at lowering AHI and improving oxygenation.[83] Side-effects of MADs include increased lower and total anterior facial height, mild temporal muscular and temporomandibular joint discomfort, dry mouth, increased salivation, tongue discomfort, and sensation of suffocation.[79]

Soft tissue surgery. Single or multi-level soft tissue surgery aims to reduce volume or tension collapse according to the site, shape, and pattern of obstruction:

1- Adenotonsillectomy. Meta-analytic review has shown tonsillectomy reduced AHI by 4.8 points and improved sleep-related quality of life, anxiety, and emotional lability.[84] Partial intracapsular tonsillectomy for pediatric SDB has been shown to be safe, reduced secondary

hemorrhage by 79%, reduced postoperative pain, and recovery time with polysomnographic improvement equal to total tonsillectomy.[85]

2- Soft palate and lateral pharyngeal wall surgery have evolved to achieve the hybrid aims of preserving mucosa, ablating adipose tissue, excising lymphoid tissue, and suspension of pharyngeal muscles to provide a stable and expanded airway.[86] Suspension procedures for lateral pharyngeal collapse include lateral pharyngoplasty, expansion sphincter pharyngoplasty, relocation pharyngoplasty, or barbed repositioning pharyngoplasty. Suspension palatoplasty is conducted for anterior–posterior palatal collapse, while concentric collapse requires a combination of pharyngeal and palatal suspension. Anterior palatoplasty, zetapalatopharyngoplasty (ZPPP), transpalatal advancement pharyngoplasty, and extended uvulopalatal flap techniques are also used to address the bulky or elongated soft palate. Systematic review (n = 2715) of palatal surgery from 2001 to 2018 showed a mean decrease in AHI from 35.66 to 13.91, a mean decrease in ESS was from 11.65 to 5.08, and an overall pooled success rate of 67.5%. Procedure-wise AHI reduction was 24.7/h for anterior palatoplasty, 19.8 for lateral/expansion pharyngoplasty, and 17.2 for uvulopalatopharyngoplasty.[87]

3- Tongue and tongue base. Lingual tonsillectomy, tongue channeling, radiofrequency of the base of tongue (RFBOT), submucosal minimally invasive lingual excision (SMILE), endoscopic coblation tongue base resection (Eco-TBR), and transoral robotic surgery for tongue base (TORS) are conducted for reducing the volume of the tongue or tongue base.[88] SMILE and RFBOT have success rates of 65% and 42%, respectively[89] with higher morbidities and complications in SMILE. Eco-TBR has a success rate of 63% when combined with ZPPP[90] and TORS has a success rate of 68%[91]

4 Lingual frenulum. Lingual frenuloplasty conducted for anterior and posterior tongue-ties, combined with MFT improves the quality of life by reducing mouth breathing (78.4%), snoring (72.9%), clenching (91.0%), and myofascial tension (77.5%) (n = 348).[92]

Skeletal surgery

Skeletal surgery aims to expand the NAC or pharyngeal airway.

NAC expansion procedures include rapid maxillary expansion (RME), surgically assisted rapid maxillary expansion (SARME), surgically assisted rapid palatal expansion (SARPE), and distraction osteogenesis maxillary expansion (DOME). Nasal obstruction tends to persist after nasal surgery when there is a high arched palate, narrow transverse maxillary width, and acute nasal angle at the pyriform aperture[20] and will benefit from NAC expansion. The selection of these procedures depends on the age and the dimensions of expansion needed. RME aims to restore a dome-shaped hard palate in children before suture fusion. After fusion, surgical osteotomies conducted in SARME and SARPE are necessary. RME expands the maxilla by an orthotic device fixed to teeth or the maxilla—increasing nasal volume, reducing nasal resistance, and enlarging the pharyngeal airway by allowing the upward and forward placement of the tongue.[93,94] RME has been shown to reduce AHI by 6.86 points in a review of 215 children of mean age 6.7 years.[95] In adults with a transversely compressed maxilla, DOME has been shown to achieve a 54% reduction in AHI, 36% reduction in ESS, and 45% increase in REM sleep time.[96]

Pharyngeal expansion procedures include genioglossus advancement (GA), hyoid myotomy and suspension (HSP), sliding genioplasty (SG), and maxillomandibular advancement (MMA).[97] GA has a success rate of 39% to 78% in a meta-analytic review with success above 60% in GA as a sole procedure.[98] MMA is indicated in severe mandibular deficiency (SNB <74°), moderate-to-severe OSA, hypopharyngeal narrowing, and failure of other forms of treatment. MMA has shown the greatest success rate (86%) and cure (43.2%) with a mean reduction in AHI from 63.9/h to 9.5 h in a meta-analytic review (n = 947.)[99]

SUMMARY

Snoring alerts us to the presence of SDB and its concomitant serious morbidities. Systematic evaluation of the patient by applying a framework of anatomic and nonanatomic phenotypes will increase the specificity of therapy. Familiarity with various modalities, their efficacies, and risks will

further tailor therapy appropriate for the patient. Management of SDB requires an integrative and multidisciplinary approach involving physicians, surgeons, dentists, and myofunctional therapists. Future research correlating treatment strategies to phenotypes is needed for furthering personalized and precision medicine.

CLINICS CARE POINTS

- A patient with snoring should be evaluated for signs and symptoms of sleep-disordered breathing
- Mouth breathing, dental abnormalities, and behavioral changes in children should alert the physician to possible sleep-disordered breathing
- Systematic examination of the upper airway should take into consideration both soft tissue and skeletal changes
- Examining for tongue range of motion should not be missed in evaluating causes for sleep-disordered breathing
- When performing a polysomnogram, level of study should be guided by comorbidities and sleep disorders suspected
- When analyzing the polysomnogram, take into consideration the low arousal threshold
- MFT should be considered in the treatment of children with sleep-disordered breathing
- In treating children with sleep-disordered breathing, integrating care with dental/oromaxillofacial input is critical

DISCLOSURE

Dr Y-Y. Yap is the principal investigator of a clinical trial in allergic rhinitis for MEDA Pharma GmbH & Co. KG (A Mylan Company) in Malaysia.

REFERENCES

1. Huang L, Quinn SJ, Ellis PD, et al. Biomechanics of snoring. Endeavour 1995;19(3):96–100.
2. Xu HJ, Jia RF, Yu H, et al. Investigation of the source of snoring sound by drug-induced sleep nasendoscopy. ORL J Otorhinolaryngol Relat Spec 2015; 77(6):359–65.
3. Moaeri S, Hildebrandt O, Cassel W, et al. Die Analyse von Schnarchen bei Patienten mit obstruktiver Schlafapnoe (OSA) anhand von Polysomnografie und LEO-Sound [analysis of snoring in patients with obstructive

sleep apnea (OSA) by Polysomnography and LEO-Sound]. Pneumologie 2020;74(8):509–14.

4. Young T, Palta M, Dempsey J, et al. The occurrence of sleep-disordered breathing among middle-aged adults. N Engl J Med 1993;328(17):1230–5.

5. Lechner M, Breeze CE, Ohayon MM, et al. Snoring and breathing pauses during sleep: interview survey of a United Kingdom population sample reveals a significant increase in the rates of sleep apnoea and obesity over the last 20 years - data from the UK sleep survey. Sleep Med 2019;54:250–6.

6. Hu FB, Willett WC, Manson JE, et al. Snoring and risk of cardiovascular disease in women. J Am Coll Cardiol 2000;35(2):308–13.

7. Senaratna CV, Perret JL, Lodge CJ, et al. Prevalence of obstructive sleep apnea in the general population: a systematic review. Sleep Med Rev 2017;34: 70–81.

8. Foley D, Ancoli-Israel S, Britz P, et al. Sleep disturbances and chronic disease in older adults: results of the 2003 National Sleep Foundation Sleep in America Survey. J Psychosom Res 2004;56(5): 497–502.

9. Zinchuk AV, Gentry MJ, Concato J, et al. Phenotypes in obstructive sleep apnea: a definition, examples and evolution of approaches. Sleep Med Rev 2017;35:113–23.

10. Carberry JC, Amatoury J, Eckert DJ. Personalized management approach for OSA. Chest 2018; 153(3):744–55.

11. Deflandre E, Gerdom A, Lamarque C, et al. Understanding pathophysiological concepts leading to obstructive apnea. Obes Surg 2018;28(8):2560–71.

12. Neelapu BC, Kharbanda OP, Sardana HK, et al. Craniofacial and upper airway morphology in adult obstructive sleep apnea patients: a systematic review and meta-analysis of cephalometric studies. Sleep Med Rev 2017;31:79–90.

13. Gupta A, Kumar R, Bhattacharya D, et al. Craniofacial and upper airway profile assessment in North Indian patients with obstructive sleep apnea. Lung India 2019;36(2):94–101.

14. Zonato AI, Bittencourt LR, Martinho FL, et al. Association of systematic head and neck physical examination with severity of obstructive sleep apnea-hypopnea syndrome. Laryngoscope 2003; 113(6):973–80.

15. Michels Dde S, Rodrigues Ada M, Nakanishi M, et al. Nasal involvement in obstructive sleep apnea syndrome. Int J Otolaryngol 2014;2014:717419.

16. Virkkula P, Maasilta P, Hytönen M, et al. Nasal obstruction and sleep-disordered breathing: the effect of supine body position on nasal measurements in snorers. Acta Otolaryngol 2003;123(5):648–54.

17. Ferris BG Jr, Mead J, Opie LH. Partitioning of respiratory flow resistance in man. J Appl Physiol 1964; 19:653–8.

18. Stuck BA, Czajkowski J, Hagner AE, et al. Changes in daytime sleepiness, quality of life, and objective sleep patterns in seasonal allergic rhinitis: a controlled clinical trial. J Allergy Clin Immunol 2004;113(4):663–8.

19. Kalpaklioğlu AF, Kavut AB, Ekici M. Allergic and nonallergic rhinitis: the threat for obstructive sleep apnea. Ann Allergy Asthma Immunol 2009;103(1): 20–5.

20. Williams R, Patel V, Chen YF, et al. The upper airway nasal complex: structural contribution to persistent nasal obstruction. Otolaryngol Head Neck Surg 2019;161(1):171–7.

21. Lenders H, Schaefer J, Pirsig W. Turbinate hypertrophy in habitual snorers and patients with obstructive sleep apnea: findings of acoustic rhinometry. Laryngoscope 1991;101(6 Pt 1):614–8.

22. Isono S, Remmers JE, Tanaka A, et al. Anatomy of pharynx in patients with obstructive sleep apnea and in normal subjects. J Appl Physiol (1985) 1997;82(4):1319–26.

23. Schwab RJ, Gupta KB, Gefter WB, et al. Upper airway and soft tissue anatomy in normal subjects and patients with sleep-disordered breathing. Significance of the lateral pharyngeal walls. Am J Respir Crit Care Med 1995;152(5 Pt 1):1673–89.

24. Dahlqvist J, Dahlqvist A, Marklund M, et al. Physical findings in the upper airways related to obstructive sleep apnea in men and women. Acta Otolaryngol 2007;127(6):623–30.

25. Mangat D, Orr WC, Smith RO. Sleep apnea, hypersomnolence, and upper airway obstruction secondary to adenotonsillar enlargement. Arch Otolaryngol 1977;103(7):383–6.

26. Weiss TM, Atanasov S, Calhoun KH. The association of tongue scalloping with obstructive sleep apnea and related sleep pathology. Otolaryngol Head Neck Surg 2005;133(6):966–71.

27. Tomooka K, Tanigawa T, Sakurai S, et al. Scalloped tongue is associated with nocturnal intermittent hypoxia among community-dwelling Japanese: the Toon Health Study. J Oral Rehabil 2017;44(8): 602–9.

28. Guilleminault C, Huseni S, Lo L. A frequent phenotype for paediatric sleep apnoea: short lingual frenulum. ERJ Open Res 2016;2(3):00043–2016.

29. Villa MP, Evangelisti M, Barreto M, et al. Short lingual frenulum as a risk factor for sleep-disordered breathing in school-age children. Sleep Med 2020; 66:119–22.

30. Brożek-Mądry E, Burska Z, Steć Z, et al. Short lingual frenulum and head-forward posture in children with the risk of obstructive sleep apnea. Int J Pediatr Otorhinolaryngol 2021;144:110699.

31. Yoon AJ, Zaghi S, Ha S, et al. Ankyloglossia as a risk factor for maxillary hypoplasia and soft palate elongation: a functional - morphological study. Orthod Craniofac Res 2017;20(4):237–44.

32. Morrell MJ, Arabi Y, Zahn B, et al. Progressive retro-palatal narrowing preceding obstructive apnea. Am J Respir Crit Care Med 1998;158(6):1974–81.

33. Sforza E, Bacon W, Weiss T, et al. Upper airway collapsibility and cephalometric variables in patients with obstructive sleep apnea. Am J Respir Crit Care Med 2000;161(2 Pt 1):347–52.

34. Squier SB, Patil SP, Schneider H, et al. Effect of end-expiratory lung volume on upper airway collapsibility in sleeping men and women. J Appl Physiol (1985) 2010;109(4):977–85.

35. McGinley BM, Schwartz AR, Schneider H, et al. Upper airway neuromuscular compensation during sleep is defective in obstructive sleep apnea. J Appl Physiol (1985) 2008;105(1):197–205.

36. Suratt PM, McTier RF, Wilhoit SC. Upper airway muscle activation is augmented in patients with obstructive sleep apnea compared with that in normal subjects. Am Rev Respir Dis 1988;137(4):889–94.

37. Eckert DJ, Lo YL, Saboisky JP, et al. Sensorimotor function of the upper-airway muscles and respiratory sensory processing in untreated obstructive sleep apnea. J Appl Physiol (1985) 2011;111(6):1644–53.

38. Deegan PC, Mulloy E, McNicholas WT. Topical oropharyngeal anesthesia in patients with obstructive sleep apnea. Am J Respir Crit Care Med 1995; 151(4):1108–12.

39. Deacon-Diaz N, Malhotra A. Inherent vs. Induced loop gain abnormalities in obstructive sleep apnea. Front Neurol 2018;9:896.

40. Subramani Y, Singh M, Wong J, et al. Understanding phenotypes of obstructive sleep apnea: applications in anesthesia, surgery, and perioperative medicine. Anesth Analg 2017;124(1):179–91.

41. Edwards BA, Eckert DJ, McSharry DG, et al. Clinical predictors of the respiratory arousal threshold in patients with obstructive sleep apnea. Am J Respir Crit Care Med 2014;190(11):1293–300.

42. Abreu RR, Rocha RL, Lamounier JA, et al. Etiology, clinical manifestations and concurrent findings in mouth-breathing children. J Pediatr (Rio J) 2008; 84(6):529–35.

43. Fitzpatrick MF, McLean H, Urton AM, et al. Effect of nasal or oral breathing route on upper airway resistance during sleep. Eur Respir J 2003;22(5):827–32.

44. McNicholas WT, Coffey M, Boyle T. Effects of nasal airflow on breathing during sleep in normal humans. Am Rev Respir Dis 1993;147(3):620–3.

45. Basner RC, Simon PM, Schwartzstein RM, et al. Breathing route influences upper airway muscle activity in awake normal adults. J Appl Physiol (1985) 1989;66(4):1766–71.

46. Izuhara Y, Matsumoto H, Nagasaki T, et al. Mouth breathing, another risk factor for asthma: the Nagahama Study. Allergy 2016;71(7):1031–6.

47. Fraga WS, Seixas VM, Santos JC, et al. Mouth breathing in children and its impact in dental malocclusion: a systematic review of observational studies. Minerva Stomatol 2018;67(3):129–38.

48. Neiva PD, Kirkwood RN, Mendes PL, et al. Postural disorders in mouth breathing children: a systematic review. Braz J Phys Ther 2018;22(1):7–19.

49. Marcus CL, Brooks LJ, Draper KA, et al. Diagnosis and management of childhood obstructive sleep apnea syndrome. Pediatrics 2012;130(3):e714–55.

50. Gipson K, Lu M, Kinane TB. Sleep-disordered breathing in children. Pediatr Rev 2019;40(1):3–13 [Erratum appears in Pediatr Rev. 2019 May;40(5):261].

51. Nieto FJ, Young TB, Lind BK, et al. Association of sleep-disordered breathing, sleep apnea, and hypertension in a large community-based study. Sleep Heart Health Study. JAMA 2000;283(14):1829–36 [Erratum appears in JAMA 2002 Oct 23-30; 288(16):1985].

52. Mokhlesi B, Finn LA, Hagen EW, et al. Obstructive sleep apnea during REM sleep and hypertension. results of the Wisconsin Sleep Cohort. Am J Respir Crit Care Med 2014;190(10):1158–67.

53. Shahar E, Whitney CW, Redline S, et al. Sleep-disordered breathing and cardiovascular disease: cross-sectional results of the Sleep Heart Health Study. Am J Respir Crit Care Med 2001;163(1):19–25.

54. Nagayoshi M, Punjabi NM, Selvin E, et al. Obstructive sleep apnea and incident type 2 diabetes. Sleep Med 2016;25:156–61.

55. Zhu X, Zhao Y. Sleep-disordered breathing and the risk of cognitive decline: a meta-analysis of 19,940 participants. Sleep Breath 2018;22(1):165–73.

56. Schwartz AR, Patil SP, Laffan AM, et al. Obesity and obstructive sleep apnea: pathogenic mechanisms and therapeutic approaches. Proc Am Thorac Soc 2008;5(2):185–92.

57. Schwab RJ, Pasirstein M, Pierson R, et al. Identification of upper airway anatomic risk factors for obstructive sleep apnea with volumetric magnetic resonance imaging. Am J Respir Crit Care Med 2003;168(5):522–30.

58. Stewart MG, Witsell DL, Smith TL, et al. Development and validation of the nasal obstruction symptom evaluation (NOSE) scale. Otolaryngol Head Neck Surg 2004;130(2):157–63.

59. Camacho M, Zaghi S, Certal V, et al. Inferior turbinate classification system, grades 1 to 4: development and validation study. Laryngoscope 2015; 125(2):296–302.

60. Locketz GD, Teo NW, Walgama E, et al. The nasal vestibular body: anatomy, clinical features, and treatment considerations. Eur Arch Otorhinolaryngol 2016;273(3):777–81.

61. Woodson BT. A method to describe the pharyngeal airway. Laryngoscope 2015;125(5):1233–8.

62. Olszewska E, Woodson BT. Palatal anatomy for sleep apnea surgery. Laryngoscope Investig Otolaryngol 2019;4(1):181–7.

63. Yoon A, Zaghi S, Weitzman R, et al. Toward a functional definition of ankyloglossia: validating current grading scales for lingual frenulum length and tongue mobility in 1052 subjects. Sleep Breath 2017;21(3):767–75.

64. Riley RW, Powell NB, Guilleminault C. Inferior mandibular osteotomy and hyoid myotomy suspension for obstructive sleep apnea: a review of 55 patients. J Oral Maxillofac Surg 1989;47(2):159–64.

65. Kezirian EJ, Hohenhorst W, de Vries N. Drug-induced sleep endoscopy: the VOTE classification. Eur Arch Otorhinolaryngol 2011;268(8):1233–6.

66. Vroegop AV, Vanderveken OM, Boudewyns AN, et al. Drug-induced sleep endoscopy in sleep-disordered breathing: report on 1,249 cases. Laryngoscope 2014;124(3):797–802.

67. Patil SP, Ayappa IA, Caples SM, et al. Treatment of adult obstructive sleep apnea with positive airway pressure: an American academy of sleep medicine systematic review, meta-analysis, and GRADE Assessment. J Clin Sleep Med 2019;15(2):301–34.

68. Martínez-García MA, Capote F, Campos-Rodríguez F, et al. Effect of CPAP on blood pressure in patients with obstructive sleep apnea and resistant hypertension: the HIPARCO randomized clinical trial. JAMA 2013;310(22):2407–15.

69. Wang G, Goebel JR, Li C, et al. Therapeutic effects of CPAP on cognitive impairments associated with OSA. J Neurol 2020;267(10):2823–8.

70. Rotenberg BW, Murariu D, Pang KP. Trends in CPAP adherence over twenty years of data collection: a flattened curve. J Otolaryngol Head Neck Surg 2016;45(1):43.

71. Camacho M, Certal V, Abdullatif J, et al. Myofunctional therapy to treat obstructive sleep apnea: a systematic review and meta-analysis. Sleep 2015; 38(5):669–75.

72. Lee SY, Guilleminault C, Chiu HY, et al. Mouth breathing, "nasal disuse," and pediatric sleep-disordered breathing. Sleep Breath 2015;19(4):1257–64.

73. Diaféria G, Santos-Silva R, Truksinas E, et al. Myofunctional therapy improves adherence to continuous positive airway pressure treatment. Sleep Breath 2017;21(2):387–95.

74. Lavigne F, Petrof BJ, Johnson JR, et al. Effect of topical corticosteroids on allergic airway inflammation and disease severity in obstructive sleep apnoea. Clin Exp Allergy 2013;43(10):1124–33.

75. Craig TJ, Teets S, Lehman EB, et al. Nasal congestion secondary to allergic rhinitis as a cause of sleep disturbance and daytime fatigue and the response to topical nasal corticosteroids. J Allergy Clin Immunol 1998;101(5):633–7.

76. Wu J, Zhao G, Li Y, et al. Apnea-hypopnea index decreased significantly after nasal surgery for obstructive sleep apnea: a meta-analysis. Medicine (Baltimore) 2017;96(5):e6008.

77. Hoffstein V, Viner S, Mateika S, et al. Treatment of obstructive sleep apnea with nasal continuous positive airway pressure. Patient compliance, perception of benefits, and side effects. Am Rev Respir Dis 1992;145(4 Pt 1):841–5.

78. Camacho M, Riaz M, Capasso R, et al. The effect of nasal surgery on continuous positive airway pressure device use and therapeutic treatment pressures: a systematic review and meta-analysis. Sleep 2015;38(2):279–86.

79. Woodson BT, Strohl KP, Soose RJ, et al. Upper airway stimulation for obstructive sleep apnea: 5-year outcomes. Otolaryngol Head Neck Surg 2018; 159(1):194–202.

80. Ng JH, Yow M. Oral appliances in the management of obstructive sleep apnea. Sleep Med Clin 2019; 14(1):109–18.

81. Deane SA, Cistulli PA, Ng AT, et al. Comparison of mandibular advancement splint and tongue stabilizing device in obstructive sleep apnea: a randomized controlled trial [published correction appears in Sleep. Sleep 2009;32(5):648–53.

82. Ramar K, Dort LC, Katz SG, et al. Clinical practice guideline for the treatment of obstructive sleep apnea and snoring with oral appliance therapy: an update for 2015. J Clin Sleep Med 2015;11(7):773–827.

83. Schwartz M, Acosta L, Hung YL, et al. Effects of CPAP and mandibular advancement device treatment in obstructive sleep apnea patients: a systematic review and meta-analysis. Sleep Breath 2018; 22(3):555–68.

84. Chinnadurai S, Jordan AK, Sathe NA, et al. Tonsillectomy for obstructive sleep-disordered breathing: a meta-analysis. Pediatrics 2017;139(2):e20163491.

85. Zhang LY, Zhong L, David M, et al. Tonsillectomy or tonsillotomy? A systematic review for paediatric sleep-disordered breathing. Int J Pediatr Otorhinolaryngol 2017;103:41–50.

86. Li HY. Palatal surgery for obstructive sleep apnea: from ablation to reconstruction. Sleep Med Clin 2019;14(1):51–8.

87. Pang KP, Plaza G, Baptista JPM, et al. Palate surgery for obstructive sleep apnea: a 17-year meta-analysis. Eur Arch Otorhinolaryngol 2018;275(7):1697–707.

88. Lin HC, Friedman M. Volumetric tongue reduction for obstructive sleep apnea. Sleep Med Clin 2019; 14(1):59–65.

89. Friedman M, Soans R, Gurpinar B, et al. Evaluation of submucosal minimally invasive lingual excision technique for treatment of obstructive sleep apnea/hypopnea syndrome. Otolaryngol Head Neck Surg 2008;139(3):378–85.

90. Lin HC, Friedman M, Chang HW, et al. Z-palatopharyngoplasty combined with endoscopic coblator open tongue base resection for severe obstructive sleep apnea/hypopnea syndrome. Otolaryngol Head Neck Surg 2014;150(6):1078–85.

91. Miller SC, Nguyen SA, Ong AA, et al. Transoral robotic base of tongue reduction for obstructive sleep apnea: a systematic review and meta-analysis. Laryngoscope 2017;127(1):258–65.

92. Zaghi S, Valcu-Pinkerton S, Jabara M, et al. Lingual frenuloplasty with myofunctional therapy: exploring safety and efficacy in 348 cases. Laryngoscope Investig Otolaryngol 2019;4(5):489–96.

93. Zambon CE, Ceccheti MM, Utumi ER, et al. Orthodontic measurements and nasal respiratory function after surgically assisted rapid maxillary expansion: an acoustic rhinometry and rhinomanometry study. Int J Oral Maxillofac Surg 2012;41(9):1120–6.

94. Iwasaki T, Saitoh I, Takemoto Y, et al. Tongue posture improvement and pharyngeal airway en-largement as secondary effects of rapid maxillary expansion: a cone-beam computed tomography study. Am J Orthod Dentofacial Orthop 2013; 143(2):235–45.

95. Machado-Júnior AJ, Zancanella E, Crespo AN. Rapid maxillary expansion and obstructive sleep apnea: a review and meta-analysis. Med Oral Patol Oral Cir Bucal 2016;21(4):e465–9.

96. Yoon A, Guilleminault C, Zaghi S, et al. Distraction Osteogenesis Maxillary Expansion (DOME) for adult obstructive sleep apnea patients with narrow maxilla and nasal floor. Sleep Med 2020;65:172–6.

97. Barrera JE. Skeletal surgery for obstructive sleep apnea. Sleep Med Clin 2018;13(4):549–58.

98. Kezirian EJ, Goldberg AN. Hypopharyngeal surgery in obstructive sleep apnea: an evidence-based medicine review. Arch Otolaryngol Head Neck Surg 2006; 132(2):206–13.

99. Holty JE, Guilleminault C. Maxillomandibular advancement for the treatment of obstructive sleep apnea: a systematic review and meta-analysis. Sleep Med Rev 2010;14(5):287–97.

Disrupted Sleep During a Pandemic

Niraj Kumar, MD, DM[a], Ravi Gupta, MD, PhD[b],*

KEYWORDS

- Sleep • SARS-CoV-2 infection • COVID-19 • Insomnia • Poor quality sleep

KEY POINTS

- Sleep disturbances may be seen in up to three-fourth of COVID-19 patients, and up to two-fifth of health care workers and general population.
- Older age, having a partner alongside, and staying in a high-income country reduced the risk of sleep disturbances.
- Younger age, female sex, financial problems and coexisting stress, anxiety, and depression enhanced the risk of sleep disturbances.
- Etiology of sleep disturbances in COVID-19 pandemic is multifactorial. Three major factors neuro-invasion by SARS-CoV-2, social factors and health-policy changes during the pandemic can be implicated as contributors.
- A close association of sleep with immunity and metabolism means identification and treatment of sleep disturbances are essential during the pandemic time.
- Support from "Telemedicine sleep clinic" along with motivating the population to manage the zeitgebers may improve sleep during the pandemic.

INTRODUCTION

A pandemic is described as a state where a disease evolves quickly, affects a significant proportion of the population, and usually spreads across geographic boundaries to involve more than one continent.[1,2] In the 21st century, the world has suffered 3 pandemics: severe acute respiratory syndrome (SARS-CoV) in 2003, Swine Flu (H1N1) in 2009, and since late 2019, COVID-19 (SARS-CoV-2).[1–3] Among them, the COVID-19 pandemic had the most marked effect on health through direct and indirect factors, by inducing physiologic alteration across systems and by paving way for economic as well as political changes in a time of scientific uncertainty.[2]

Sleep is one of the important physiologic activities performed by all animal species. Contrary to prevalent belief of many, sleep is no longer considered as a period of inactivity by the sleep scientific community. Indeed, it is associated with several important functions required for a healthy life—rejuvenation, memory consolidation, modulation of immune function, and regulation of hormonal secretion.[4,5] The pandemic has affected sleep in different ways. For a considerable proportion of the population, sleep has worsened in terms of quality, duration, and timing, but for a small proportion, it has improved.[6] Sleep was affected by several factors during the COVID-19 pandemic. Unprecedented lockdowns limited zeitgebers (eg, physical activity, exposure to daylight, social rhythm, screen exposure, time of food intake) that regulate the sleep-wake cycle. Studies have also shown that a sizable number of people experience distress associated with uncertainties regarding

Credit Lines: All the illustrations (figures and tables) are drawn/prepared by the authors; hence, permission from a third party is not required.

[a] Department of Neurology, Division of Sleep Medicine, All India Institute of Medical Sciences, Rishikesh 249203, India; [b] Department of Psychiatry, Division of Sleep Medicine, All India Institute of Medical Sciences, Rishikesh 249203, India

* Corresponding author. Department of Psychiatry and Division of Sleep Medicine, All India Institute of Medical Sciences, Rishikesh 249203, India.

E-mail address: sleepdoc.ravi@gmail.com

Sleep Med Clin 17 (2022) 41–52
https://doi.org/10.1016/j.jsmc.2021.10.006
1556-407X/22/© 2021 Elsevier Inc. All rights reserved.

the course of treatment and outcome of SARS-CoV-2 infection, as well as their employment.[7] Together, these issues led to changes in sleep duration, timing, and quality in *vulnerable* individuals.[7] For others, the lockdown was a respite that increased the sleep duration and improved sleep quality as suggested by reduction of social jet lag.[8,9]

Though the impact of pandemics on sleep has also been studied, it has been most extensively researched during the current COVID-19 pandemic. This article will present the available literature and will be divided into the following sections for better understanding.

1. Magnitude of sleep disturbances during the pandemic
2. Determinants and pathophysiology of sleep disturbances during COVID-19 pandemic
3. Long-term perspectives of sleep disturbances
4. Why is there a need to pay attention to sleep disorders during pandemics
5. Management of sleep disturbances during a pandemic

MAGNITUDE OF SLEEP DISTURBANCES DURING THE PANDEMIC

Sleep disturbances during pandemics have been reported across different age groups and in a variety of populations ranging from the general population and front-line workers to hospitalized and quarantined patients with SARS-CoV-2 infection. Available studies focused on the assessment of sleep quality, sleep-wake schedule, and insomnia.

The magnitude of sleep problems reported in studies is influenced by several factors: time at which the problem was assessed (lockdown vs after unlocking), age, gender, comorbidity, and medication history of subjects. It has been reported that detrimental changes in sleep pattern during early lockdown tend to remain the same unless early intervention is provided.[10] Choice of questionnaires and measures used to assess sleep also affected the results across studies. For example, a higher prevalence of poor sleep quality has been reported from the studies using standardized measures of sleep like the Pittsburgh Sleep Quality Index (PSQI) compared with studies using other scales and investigator-developed measurements.[11] Cut-off scores of the questionnaires also influenced the outcomes; the cut-off for the PSQI was higher than standard in some of the studies that could have resulted in lower prevalence.[12] A summary of the available meta-analysis which addressed the prevalence of sleep disturbances during the COVID-19 pandemic is presented in **Table 1**.

Sleep Quality

Among adults

Sleep health includes 6 measures, namely regularity of sleep-wake schedule, duration of sleep, timing of sleep and wake, satisfaction with sleep, sleep efficiency, and daytime alertness. These are all indirect measures of sleep quality.[17] Poor sleep health was reported by nearly one-fourth to half of the adult participants ranging between 18 and 94 years of age.[9,17] There was a geographic variation in sleep health, with poorer sleep health among residents of Latin American and Caribbean countries compared with residents of North America, Europe, and Central Asia.[17] Owing to geographic variation, pooled analysis would provide better estimates of disturbed sleep among the general population. A systematic review reported that in the general population, nearly one-third had reported disturbed sleep.[11]

In a pooled analysis of sleep using questionnaires, sleep disturbance was shown to be higher among health care workers (HCWs) at nearly 40%.[11,16] Similar to the general population, geographic variation of sleep disturbance was also noted among HCWs; it was lower in China compared with other countries like Bahrain and Iraq.[16] Contrary to intuitive deduction, it is difficult to reliably comment whether prevalence has actually increased among HCW during the pandemic as it appeared comparable to pre-pandemic time at least by one at study group.[11]

A systematic review of cross-sectional studies reported that sleep quality was poor during the pandemic, not only in HCWs (irrespective of their engagement in the management of COVID-19 patients during the pandemic) but also among nonhospitalized individuals (irrespective of the status of SARS-CoV-2 infection).[18] Interestingly, in most of the studies, poor sleep quality was reported despite spending longer time in bed.[18] This is a situation similar to paradoxic insomnia wherein despite an adequate sleep duration, sleep is still nonrefreshing, perhaps owing to increased cortical activation.[19]

Patients with SARS-CoV-2 infection make the largest proportion of the group in which sleep quality was poor during pandemic (nearly three-fourth reported).[11] This is in contrast to another meta-analysis, which reported that only 34% of patients having SARS-CoV-2 infection had disturbed sleep or poor quality sleep.[12] In the latter paper, most of the studies were from China, whereas the earlier paper represented better global prevalence because it included studies from various countries.

Contrary to reports of poor or worsening sleep quality in most studies, a minority of the population

Table 1
Prevalence of sleep disturbances during COVID-19 pandemic across meta-analyses

S.N.	Authors	Population and Time of Study	Assessment Measures	Pooled Prevalence	Limitations
1.	Jahrami et al,[11] 2021	• Adults from the general population • Patients having SARS-CoV-2 infection • Health care workers	• Researcher developed • Athens Insomnia Scale • PSQI • Insomnia Severity Index	35.7%	• Different measures used to assess sleep quality and quantity • Assessment of sleep disturbance not the primary focus in 20% of the studies
2.	Deng et al,[12] 2021	COVID-19 patients	• Researcher developed • PSQI • Insomnia Severity Index • Clinical interview	34%	• Most studies were from China • Significant heterogeneity among studies • Cut-off for PSQI was 16–21
3.	Panda et al,[13] 2021	Children with and without psychiatric disorders	Not mentioned for sleep disorders	21.3%	• Questionnaire-based assessment • Timing of data gathering in relation to pandemic not clear
4.	Pappa et al,[14] 2020	Health care workers	• Insomnia Severity Index • Athens Insomnia Scale • PSQI	34%	Most studies were from China
5.	Salari et al,[15] 2020	Nurses and physicians	• Insomnia Severity Index • Athens Insomnia Scale • PSQI	Nurses: 35% Physicians: 42%	Most studies were from China
6.	Marvaldi et al,[16] 2021	Health care workers	• Insomnia Severity Index • PSQI	44%	Most studies were from China

(6%) reported improvement of sleep during the pandemic.[6] With one study reporting nearly a quarter of subjects having improvement in sleep quality during the lockdown irrespective of the total sleep time at night.[9]

Taken altogether, the available data show that geographic variation exists among subjects reporting poor sleep quality both in the general population and in patients suffering from SARS-CoV-2 infection. These factors could also emphasize the role of genetics in their vulnerability (eg, MEIS1 gene has been found to be associated with insomnia, MEIS1 and BTBD-9 have been found to increase the risk for restless legs syndrome, etc.) to develop sleep disturbances in association with environmental factors.[7]

Among children and adolescents
Poor and worsening quality of sleep was observed among nonhospitalized children and adolescents from Spain and India.[20,21] Dutta and colleagues reported worsening of sleep among a third of children

in India.[21] However, sleep quality did not take a downhill course throughout the pandemic. It seemed to worsen in the initial phase of lockdown and thereafter remained stable.[10] And compared with adults, a greater proportion of children (43%) reported deeper sleep during the lockdown.[21]

Sleep-Wake Schedule

Among adults
Two major shifts in the sleep-wake schedule were reported during the COVID-19 pandemic—delayed sleep phase and extension of sleep time. A shift to a later bedtime and later wake time was reported by nearly 50% to 60% of the adult population in an online survey conducted across 59 countries.[17] However, figures vary across studies and a study from India reported that only a third of the subjects had delayed sleep-wake schedules.[9] In Canada, 63% of subjects had earlier bedtime and later wake time during the lockdown, whereas only 2% of the population

reported the same from India.[6,9] This suggested an extension of bedtime that had occurred during the pandemic in some of the population. Extension of sleep resulted in reduction of social jet lag during lockdowns and maintained consistent circadian rhythm across weeks.[8]

Difficulty in sleep initiation (approximately 39%) and in maintaining sleep (32%) was reported by the adult population during the COVID-19 pandemic.[17] Although difficulty in sleep initiation resulted in delayed awakening, prominent problems in sleep maintenance and early morning awakenings resulted in reduced total sleep time.[6]

Among children and adolescents

There is no meta-analysis available on sleep-wake schedule for this population. Findings across different individual studies, on the other hand, appeared to contradict one another. One study reported a change to a later bedtime and wake time on weekdays, but not on weekends (which were already delayed even before lockdown).[21] The delayed bedtime and delayed wake time were reported among children aged 3 to 16 years.[22,23] This could be related to the prolongation of sleep-onset latency, both on weekdays and weekends.[21,23] Similarly, the frequency of napping also increased after lockdown in one study, whereas reduced in another.[21,23] Interestingly, the sleep-wake changes did not develop to a free-running type of schedule. Rather, it worsened for an initial period after lockdown and remained stable thereafter.[10]

Duration of Sleep

Among adults

On average, a total sleep duration of 7 hours was reported among adults during the pandemic.[6,17] Those who used to sleep shorter than 6 to 8 hours before pandemic had reduced sleep duration pandemic, whereas those who usually slept for 6 to 8 hours during pre-pandemic period, did not report any change in either their sleep duration or had an increase in time spent asleep.[17]

Among children and adolescents

In children aged 3 to 18 years, there was an increase in the total sleep time.[13,23] In one study, half of the children were sleeping 12 hours a day, and only one-fourth were sleeping less than 8 hours a day.[22] Being cross-sectional in design, this study was not able to comment on the change in sleep duration. There was an increase in total sleep time on weekdays, but there was no change on weekends reported after lockdown.[21] This also varies geographically, with a greater change in Italy compared with Spain.[24]

Groupings Based on Change in Sleep-Wake Schedule

Based on the change in sleep-wake schedule during pandemic, 3 populations were identified in one study—extended time in bed (63% subjects), reduced time in bed (13%), and delayed sleep (24%).[6] Fewer work responsibilities and working from home resulted in delayed sleep.[6] Perhaps these people were able to follow their own sleep-wake schedules because of lack of compulsion to adhere to a structured routine. Gupta and colleagues[9] identified 3 groups in a population based survey—reduced sleep duration (16%), extended sleep duration (18%), and participants where total sleep time remained unchanged (66%). Similar to results of above mentioned study, nearly equal proportion of participants (28%) in this study fell into the "delayed sleep" category. Subjects in the reduced sleep group reported prolonged sleep onset latency and depressive features.[9] Thus, the available data suggest that sleep schedule vary across studies. The lower prevalence in the Gupta and colleagues study could be related to the inclusion of HCWs in the study population.[9] These findings also emphasize the role of social factors and structured routine as a zeitgeber.[25]

Sleep Disorders During the Lockdown

Among healthy adults, the prevalence of insomnia during lockdown appeared to remain similar to the prelockdown period.[9] Yet sleep physicians report an increase in the number of patients seeking help for insomnia and delayed sleep-wake phase sleep disorders.[26] Underlying factors are not known but could be related to the availability of teleconsultation facilities, ability to spare time for health issues, and increased awareness of health issues in view of the prevailing situation.

Contrary to adults, sleep disorders increased among children. There was an increase in difficulty falling asleep, night-time awakenings, nightmares, sleep terrors, and excessive daytime sleepiness in the preadolescent age group.[23]

DETERMINANTS AND PATHOPHYSIOLOGY OF SLEEP DISTURBANCES

Several factors were responsible for clinically significant sleep disturbances during the pandemic (**Table 2**). Interestingly, the presence of anxiety (threat perception) among parents lessened the sleep time of children, suggesting the role of shared genes as well as the environment in the occurrence of anxiety.[24]

Table 2
Protective and detrimental factors related to sleep

Protective	Detrimental
Older age[17]	Younger age[11]
Having a partner[17]	Good sleep before pandemic[6]
Living in high-income countries[17]	Women[6]
	Being employed[6]
	Financial problems[17]
	Family responsibilities[6]
	Chronic diseases[6]
	Stress and anxiety[6,17,24]
	Depression[6,17]
	Increased alcohol consumption[6,17]
	Stricter lockdown[17]
	Longer screen time[21,23]
	Physical inactivity in previously active persons[27]

Directly Related to the Illness

COVID-19 can cause sleep disruption due to nervous system invasion or systemic (non-neural) invasion along with cytokine storm (**Fig. 1**).

Nervous system invasion

Several potential pathways of neuro-invasion have been suggested for SARS-CoV-2. It may have a trans-synaptic spread where the virus retrogradely travels to the CNS after entering the peripheral nerve terminals of its primary target organs viz., oronasal mucosa and lungs. From nasal mucosa, it may spread through cribriform plate and olfactory pathways to reach the cerebral cortex. SARS-CoV-2 can also enter CNS by crossing the blood-brain barrier (BBB) through one of the two routes-either by infecting and traveling across vascular endothelium or by infecting leukocytes, which then cross the BBB ("Trojan Horse"

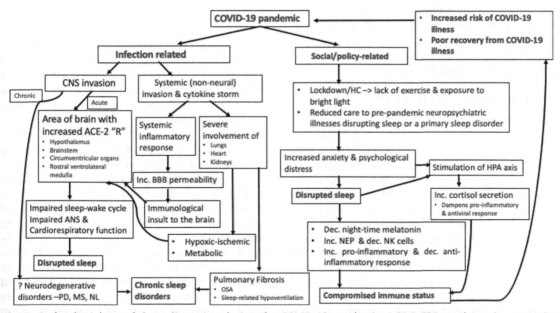

Fig. 1. Pathophysiology of sleep disruption during the COVID-19 pandemic. ACE-2 "R", angiotensin-converting enzyme-2 receptor; ANS, autonomic nervous system; BBB, blood-brain barrier; CNS, central nervous system; COVID-19, coronavirus disease 2019; Dec., decreased; HC, home confinement; HPA, hypothalamic-pituitary-adrenal axis; Inc., increased; MS, multiple sclerosis; NEP, norepinephrine; NK cells, natural killer cells; NL, narcolepsy; OSA, obstructive sleep apnea; PD, Parkinson disease.

mechanism).[28] Once inside the brain, SARS-CoV-2 invades tissues with ACE-2 receptors including the frontotemporal cortex, circumventricular organs, thalamus, and brainstem involving the rostral ventrolateral medulla among others.[28,29] ACE-2 expression has also been reported in the hypothalamus and pituitary gland.[30] Involvement of the hypothalamus and the brainstem may result in impairment of sleep-wake cycle regulation and dysautonomia with cardiorespiratory dysfunction, thereby, resulting in poor sleep quality presenting as insomnia and sleep-disordered breathing.[31]

Systemic invasion

Although the primary involved organ in SARS-CoV-2 is the lungs, other organs including the heart and kidneys may also be infected causing cardiorespiratory and metabolic derangements. The former may result in hypoxic-ischemic events and the latter causes metabolic encephalopathy.[28] In addition, a systemic inflammatory response may increase the BBB permeability, thereby, predisposing the brain to immunologic insult from a cytokine storm, which may precipitate neuropsychiatric features.[28,32] This, in turn, may result in sleep disruption.

In addition, the possibility of pulmonary fibrosis after severe COVID pneumonia may result in OSA and sleep-related hypoventilation as a long-term post-COVID complication.[33] Systemic hyperinflammation leading to deranged immunity in COVID-19 may lead to BBB compromise and involvement of the gut-brain axis, thereby, raising the possibility of developing chronic neuroinflammatory and neurodegenerative disorders such as Parkinson disease, multiple sclerosis, narcolepsy, and associated sleep disorders.[34]

Indirectly Related to COVID-19

Social factors

During the pandemic, COVID-19 patients are confined in hospitals or quarantined in their homes/facilities. Most of the noninfected population remain restricted in their homes. COVID-19 has been linked to increased anxiety and psychological distress in affected patients. Psychological distress may result from physical discomfort, hospitalization in an unknown scenario among unacquainted caregivers, and uncertainty in the course of illness.[32,35,36] In fact, disturbed mental health and long-term neuropsychiatric sequelae may follow COVID-19 illness in vulnerable patients.[37] Stress and mental ill-health, in turn, disrupt sleep.[38] Noninfected population also reports significant anxiety, stress, and sleep disruption.[9,35,39,40] This may be due to disrupted circadian rhythm owing to lack of exposure to bright light, change in sleep-wake pattern, reduced physical exercise, unpredictability regarding health and economic condition in the general population confined at home.[41]

Relation to changes in health policies

From the onset of this pandemic, focus of the health system shifted toward COVID-19, and rightly so. But this significantly impacted the availability of medical care for patients suffering from other medical disorders including those with prepandemic neuropsychiatric illnesses.[31] In fact, patients with prepandemic neuropsychiatric illnesses such as Parkinson disease reported significant sleep disturbances.[42] The pandemic significantly affected the "Sleep Medicine" practice and influenced care of patients having sleep disorders even before the pandemic.[43] A significant reduction in laboratory-based continuous positive airway pressure or bilevel positive airway pressure (PAP) titration studies was reported.[43] Owing to the risk of aerosol generation, the use of PAP was even discouraged.[44] These changes in health policies could have resulted in increased anxiety and psychological distress and contributed to further worsening of sleep in patients with preexisting pre sleep disorders.

Increased anxiety and psychological distress activate the hypothalamus-pituitary-adrenal axis and stimulate cortisol secretion. Sleep disruption resulting from increased anxiety and psychological distress may further worsen stress, forming a vicious cycle between stress and sleep disruption.[45] The resulting hypercortisolism dampens the proinflammatory pathways and antiviral immunity suffers. Increased norepinephrine levels in sleep-disrupted patients suppress natural killer cells, thereby, further compromising the immune status.[46–48] Reduced night-time melatonin, observed in patients with disrupted sleep, may deprive the patient of its anti-inflammatory, antioxidant, and immunomodulatory properties, thereby increasing risk of infection there.[49,50]

Thus, the etiology of sleep disturbances during COVID-19 appears multifactorial. If left unattended, sleep deprivation may result in enhanced functioning of proinflammatory cytokines including interleukin (IL)-1, IL-6, and tumor necrosis factor-alpha; and suppression of anti-inflammatory cytokines including IL-10.[51,52] This may predispose patients to inflammatory disorders by enhancing the expression of proinflammatory genes.[52] By affecting antioxidant enzymes, long-term sleep deprivation may also precipitate oxidative stress.[53] Unmanaged sleep abnormalities in the general population increase the risk of COVID-19 and can negatively influence the recovery of those infected. Thus, sleep disruption during the pandemic appears to play an essential role in the propagation of COVID-19.

Effect of pandemic on patients with existing sleep disorders

There is an increase in the risk of contracting COVID-19 infection among patients with sleep disorders, especially OSA. The pandemic led to the closure of sleep medicine facilities and a sharp decline in available services, leaving patients with sleep disorders without treatment.[26,43,54,55] In time, many centers chose to serve their patients via telemedicine and provided limited treatment.[26,43,55] The pandemic has become a boon for the development of telemedicine facilities and many physicians prefer to continue even after the pandemic is over.[26] This could reduce the cost of care for patients, especially indirect costs incurred toward the treatment.

LONG-TERM PERSPECTIVES OF SLEEP DISORDERS IN VIEW OF PANDEMIC

As discussed in the pathophysiology section, SARS-CoV-2 infection may leave a permanent scar in the form of neuropsychiatric sequela. Rogers and colleagues[37] reported that 12% of subjects reported insomnia as long as 24 months after recovery from SARS and MERS infection. Insomnia has been reported in nearly one-third of the patients even after months of recovery from SARS-CoV-2 infection.[56]

Literature derived from SARS infection shows that nearly a quarter of patients suffer from anxiety, depressive feelings, and post-traumatic stress disorder (PTSD) during acute infection until after 6 months.[57] These disorders are frequently associated with disturbed sleep, especially insomnia. Other sleep disorders, for example, restless legs syndrome, parasomnia may arise in association with psychotropics used for the treatment of these disorders. HCWs were likewise found to have anxiety, depressive features, and PTSD during and after the SARS pandemic.[57] Hence, there is a need to screen HCWs for sleep disturbances and sleep disorders even after the COVID-19 pandemic is over.

WHY IS THERE A NEED TO PAY ATTENTION TO SLEEP DISORDERS DURING PANDEMICS?

Several factors emphasize the need to pay attention to sleep. First, systemic inflammatory changes and sleep disturbances run in a vicious cycle. To interrupt it, attention should be paid to reduce systemic inflammation as well as restore good quality and optimal sleep. Second, vaccination is considered a major weapon against the SARS-COV-2 infection. Sleep deprivation reduces the immune response to vaccines[58] and optimal duration of sleep is important for mounting an adequate immunologic response after vaccination. However, data regarding sleep quality are not available.[58] Third, timing of vaccination is important as immune response follows a circadian pattern, being greater if vaccine is given in the morning hours.[58] Fourth, subjects with OSA are at higher risk for complications from SARS-COV-2 infection such as admission to intensive care units and death.[54,59] It is a known fact that obesity is a risk factor for OSA. Increased production of cytokines, reduced adiponectin, endothelial dysfunction, activation of prothrombotic cascade, ectopic lipid in alveolar type 2 cells, and insulin resistance have been proposed to worsen course of SARS-COV-2 infection among these individuals.[60] OSA has been found to worsen many of these parameters, adding the risk reported in earlier studies.

MANAGEMENT OF SLEEP DISTURBANCES AND SLEEP DISORDERS

In response to the COVID-19 pandemic, several medical societies have proposed guidelines to improve sleep for patients, strategies to manage sleep disorders, and continue sleep-related services for patients during the lockdown. **Table 3** summarizes these published guidelines.

Sleep disturbances during the lockdown were multifactorial and occurred only in predisposed subjects, as already discussed. As sleep-wake schedules have changed in a large proportion of the population, it has been advised that maintenance of proper routine and sleep hygiene practices needs to be followed even during lockdown.[68] Timing of intervention is important. Early intervention is more useful for prevention and can be achieved through dissemination of educational information, whereas intervention initiated in the later period needs to be more structured and individualized.[10]

Social jet lag was shown to be reduced during the lockdown among subjects who discontinued work or were working from home.[8] There is a need to educate the population regarding the importance of adequate sleep duration and manage work schedules irrespective of prevailing situations. This will help lessen sleep deprivation and boost immunity. Time saved from commuting and reduced workload may be used to increase daylight exposure, exercise, and social communication, and cultivate hobbies. All these factors are known to improve sleep quality.[39,69]

Table 3
Published literature for sleep medicine practice during the pandemic

S.N.	Title	Society	Issues Addressed
1.	Considerations for the practice of sleep medicine during COVID-19[61]	American Academy of Sleep Medicine	• COVID-19 testing before sleep study • Home Sleep Apnea Test (HSAT) and In-lab testing • PAP therapy • Mitigating risk of personnel, facility, and equipment
2.	Dealing with sleep problems during home confinement due to the COVID-19 outbreak: Practical recommendations from a task force of the European CBT-I Academy[39]	European CBT-I Academy	Nonpharmacological methods for: • Improving sleep during home confinement • Recommendations for women and children • Recommendations for health care workers and those with increased burden • Medications to improve sleep
3.	Guidelines of the Indian Society for Sleep Research (ISSR) for Practice of Sleep Medicine during COVID-19[62]	Indian Society for Sleep Research (ISSR)	• Telemedicine consultation: • who can be provided tele-consultation, methods, advantages and limitations, legal issues, online prescriptions • Sleep study during COVID-19: safety of staff and patients, indications for HSAT and in-lab testing • PAP therapy during COVID-19: Current PAP users, titration methods at home and in-laboratory, temporary auto-PAP therapy in high-risk patients
4.	Sleep laboratories reopening and COVID-19: a European perspective[63]	European Respiratory Society and National Societies	• Conducting diagnostic study for OSA • Protocol for titration study • Protocol for patients already using PAP • Recommendation for pediatric sleep studies
5.	The Society of Behavioral Sleep Medicine (SBSM) COVID-19 Task Force: Objectives and Summary Recommendations for Managing Sleep during a Pandemic[64]	Society of Behavioral Sleep Medicine	• Managing acute insomnia • Managing irregular/delayed sleep-wake schedule • Managing nightmares • Considerations for children and elders
6.	Helping Canadian health care providers to optimize Sleep Disordered Breathing management for their patients during the COVID-19 pandemic[65]	Canadian Thoracic Society	• Outpatients visit and sleep study • Patients using PAP at home • Patients with OSA using PAP while admitted to hospital • Newly diagnosed OSA patients where PAP is required

(continued on next page)

Table 3 *(continued)*			
S.N.	**Title**	**Society**	**Issues Addressed**
7.	Sleep Breathing Disorders in the COVID-19 Era: Italian Thoracic Society Organizational Models for a Correct Approach to Diagnosis and Treatment[66]	Italian Thoracic Society	• Diagnostic Sleep Study • Initiation of PAP therapy • Follow-up of patients with OSA
8.	Restoring Pulmonary and Sleep Services as the COVID-19 Pandemic Lessens. From an Association of Pulmonary, Critical Care, and Sleep Division Directors and American Thoracic Society-coordinated Task Force[67]	Association of Pulmonary, Critical Care, and Sleep Division Directors American Thoracic Society	• Guidelines for resuming outpatient services • Polysomnography services • Other respiratory services like bronchoscopy, pulmonary function testing

As OSA is a risk factor, at least for contracting SARS-CoV-2 infection with potentially poor outcomes, patients should be screened for OSA. The 5 items of the Sleep Symptoms Scale can be used and high-risk patients may be advised home sleep apnea testing (HSAT), attended polysomnography, mitigation strategies, or titration with PAP device as per prevailing guidelines.[61,70] Exercise has also been found to improve the apnea-hypopnea index.[69] Hence, this may be advised to high-risk persons.

Reduction of exposure to negative information, particularly related to COVID-19, scheduling time to introspect and identify stress, sharing the stress with members of the family to identify possible solutions, reduction and sharing of burden for daily chores, and engagement in relaxing activities before bedtime have been recommended to improve sleep.[39]

Though cognitive behavior therapy for insomnia is recommended as the first-line therapy, its availability is an issue.[39,71] In such cases, hypnotic medications may be given according to available guidelines.[71,72]

SUMMARY

During the COVID-19 pandemic, sleep disturbance increased in selected groups. Owing to the closure of sleep medicine services, patients had limited access to appropriate care and telemedicine became a viable alternative. Several sleep societies developed guidelines to improve sleep health in different populations and to adapt the practice of sleep medicine during the pandemic. Sleep disturbances were also shown to have a multifactorial origin. Evidence from basic sciences and clinical literature suggests that sleep disturbances can run a chronic course, and there

is a need to educate people about sleep disturbances during the pandemic. Lastly, patients suffering from SARS-CoV-2 infection should also be screened and treated for sleep disorders during the acute phase and after recovery.

CLINICS CARE POINTS

- All patients should be screened for sleep quality and sleep patterns during the pandemic time
- Knowledge about sleep hygiene rules should be offered to all patients
- Patients with existing sleep disorders or at high risk for sleep disorders should be referred to sleep physicians for the management of sleep disorders

DISCLOSURE

The authors have nothing to disclose.

REFERENCES

1. Swetha G, Eashwar VMA, Gopalakrishnan S. Epidemics and pandemics in India throughout history: a review article. Indian J Public Health Res Dev 2019;10(8).
2. Huremović D. Brief history of pandemics (pandemics throughout history). Psychiatry of pandemics: A Mental Health Response to Infection Outbreak, 2019. Cham, Switzerland: Springer Nature; 2019. p. 7–35.
3. Cherry JD, Krogstad P. SARS: The first pandemic of the 21st century. Pediatr Res 2004;56(1):1–5.

4. Reinke H, Asher G. Crosstalk between metabolism and circadian clocks. Nat Rev Mol Cell Biol 2019; 20(4):227–41.

5. Pocivavsek A, Rowland LM. Basic neuroscience illuminates causal relationship between sleep and memory: translating to schizophrenia. Schizophr Bull 2018;44(1):7–14.

6. Robillard R, Dion K, Pennestri MH, et al. Profiles of sleep changes during the COVID-19 pandemic: demographic, behavioural and psychological factors. J Sleep Res 2021;30(1):e13231.

7. Morin CM, Carrier J, Bastien C, et al. Sleep and circadian rhythm in response to the COVID-19 pandemic. Can J Public Health 2020;111(5):654–7.

8. Leone MJ, Sigman M, Golombek DA. Effects of lockdown on human sleep and chronotype during the COVID-19 pandemic. Curr Biol 2020;30(16):R930–1.

9. Gupta R, Grover S, Basu A, et al. Changes in sleep pattern and sleep quality during COVID-19 lockdown. Indian J Psychiatry 2020;62(4):370–8.

10. Dellagiulia A, Lionetti F, Fasolo M, et al. Early impact of COVID-19 lockdown on children's sleep: a 4-week longitudinal study. J Clin Sleep Med 2020;16(9): 1639–40.

11. Jahrami H, BaHammam AS, Bragazzi NL, et al. Sleep problems during the COVID-19 pandemic by population: a systematic review and meta-analysis. J Clin Sleep Med 2021;17(2):299–313.

12. Deng J, Zhou F, Hou W, et al. The prevalence of depression, anxiety, and sleep disturbances in COVID-19 patients: a meta-analysis. Ann N Y Acad Sci 2021;1486(1):90–111.

13. Panda PK, Gupta J, Chowdhury SR, et al. Psychological and behavioral impact of lockdown and quarantine measures for COVID-19 pandemic on children, adolescents and caregivers: a systematic review and meta-analysis. J Trop Pediatr 2021; 67(1):fmaa122.

14. Pappa S, Ntella V, Giannakas T, et al. Prevalence of depression, anxiety, and insomnia among healthcare workers during the COVID-19 pandemic: a systematic review and meta-analysis. Brain Behav Immun 2020;88:901–7.

15. Salari N, Khazaie H, Hosseinian-Far A, et al. The prevalence of sleep disturbances among physicians and nurses facing the COVID-19 patients: a systematic review and meta-analysis. Global Health 2020; 16(1):92.

16. Marvaldi M, Mallet J, Dubertret C, et al. Anxiety, depression, trauma-related, and sleep disorders among healthcare workers during the COVID-19 pandemic: a systematic review and meta-analysis. Neurosci Biobehav Rev 2021;126:252–64.

17. Yuksel D, Mckee GB, Perrin PB, et al. Sleeping when the world locks down: correlates of sleep health during the COVID-19 pandemic across 59 countries. Sleep Health 2021;7(2):134–42.

18. Souza LFF, Paineiras-Domingos LL, Melo-Oliveira MES, et al. The impact of COVID-19 pandemic in the quality of sleep by Pittsburgh Sleep Quality Index: a systematic review. Cien Saude Colet 2021;26(4):1457–66.

19. Rezaie L, Fobian AD, McCall WV, et al. Paradoxical insomnia and subjective-objective sleep discrepancy: a review. Sleep Med Rev 2018;40:196–202.

20. Lavigne-Cerván R, Costa-López B, Juárez-Ruiz De Mier R, et al. Consequences of COVID-19 confinement on anxiety, sleep and executive functions of children and adolescents in Spain. Front Psychol 2021;12:565516.

21. Dutta K, Mukherjee R, Sen D, et al. Effect of COVID-19 lockdown on sleep behavior and screen exposure time: an observational study among Indian school children. Biol Rhythm Res 2020;1–12.

22. Ranjbar K, Hosseinpour H, Shahriarirad R, et al. Students' attitude and sleep pattern during school closure following COVID-19 pandemic quarantine: a web-based survey in south of Iran. Environ Health Prev Med 2021;26(1):33.

23. Bruni O, Malorgio E, Doria M, et al. Changes in sleep patterns and disturbances in children and adolescents in Italy during the Covid-19 outbreak. Sleep Med 2021. S1389-9457(21)00094-0.

24. Orgilés M, Morales A, Delvecchio E, et al. Immediate psychological effects of the COVID-19 quarantine in youth from Italy and Spain. Front Psychol 2020;11: 579038.

25. Mistlberger R, Skene D. Social influences on mammalian circadian rhythms: animal and human studies. Biol Rev Camb Philos Soc 2004;79(3): 533–56.

26. Kanchan S, Saini LK, Daga R, et al. Status of the practice of sleep medicine in India during COVID-19 pandemic. J Clin Sleep Med 2021;17(6):1229–35.

27. Martínez-De-Quel Ó, Suárez-Iglesias D, López-Flores M, et al. Physical activity, dietary habits and sleep quality before and during COVID-19 lockdown: a longitudinal study. Appetite 2021;158: 105019.

28. Desai I, Manchanda R, Kumar N, et al. Neurological manifestations of coronavirus disease 2019: exploring past to understand present. Neurol Sci 2021;42(3):773–85.

29. Tremblay ME, Madore C, Bordeleau M, et al. Neuropathobiology of COVID-19: the role for glia. Front Cell Neurosci 2020;14:592214.

30. Pal R, Banerjee M. COVID-19 and the endocrine system: exploring the unexplored. J Endocrinol Invest 2020;43(7):1027–31.

31. Gupta R, Pandi-Perumal SR. SARS-CoV-2 infection: paving way for sleep disorders in long term. Sleep Vigil 2021;17:1–2.

32. Guo Q, Zheng Y, Shi J, et al. Immediate psychological distress in quarantined patients with COVID-19

and its association with peripheral inflammation: a mixed-method study. Brain Behav Immun 2020; 88(January):17–27.

33. Miller MA, Cappuccio FP. A systematic review of COVID-19 and obstructive sleep apnoea. Sleep Med Rev 2021;55:101382.

34. Schirinzi T, Landi D, Liguori C. COVID-19: dealing with a potential risk factor for chronic neurological disorders. J Neurol 2021;268(4):1171–8.

35. Wu KK, Chan SK, Ma TM. Posttraumatic stress, anxiety, and depression in survivors of severe acute respiratory syndrome (SARS). J Trauma Stress 2005; 18(1):39–42.

36. Silverstone PH. Prevalence of psychiatric disorders in medical inpatients. J Nerv Ment Dis 1996;184(1): 43–51.

37. Rogers JP, Chesney E, Oliver D, et al. Psychiatric and neuropsychiatric presentations associated with severe coronavirus infections: a systematic review and meta-analysis with comparison to the COVID-19 pandemic. Lancet Psychiatry 2020;7(7):611–27.

38. Van Reeth O, Weibel L, Spiegel K, et al. Interactions between stress and sleep: from basic research to clinical situations. Sleep Med Rev 2000;4(2):201–19.

39. Altena E, Baglioni C, Espie CA, et al. Dealing with sleep problems during home confinement due to the COVID-19 outbreak: practical recommendations from a task force of the European CBT-I Academy. J Sleep Res 2020;29(4):e13052.

40. Voitsidis P, Gliatas I, Bairachtari V, et al. Insomnia during the COVID-19 pandemic in a Greek population. Psychiatry Res 2020;289:113076.

41. de Sousa Martins e Silva E, Ono BHVS, Souza JC. Sleep and immunity in times of COVID-19. Rev Assoc Med Bras (1992) 2020;66(Suppl 2):143–7.

42. Kumar N, Gupta R, Kumar H, et al. Impact of home confinement during COVID-19 pandemic on Parkinson's disease. Parkinsonism Relat Disord 2020;80: 32–4.

43. Grote L, Mcnicholas WT, Hedner J. Sleep apnoea management in Europe during the COVID-19 pandemic: data from the European sleep apnoea database (ESADA). Eur Respir J 2020;55(6): 2001323.

44. Barker J, Oyefeso O, Koeckerling D, et al. COVID-19: community CPAP and NIV should be stopped unless medically necessary to support life. Thorax 2020;75(5):367.

45. Åkerstedt T. Psychosocial stress and impaired sleep. Scand J Work Environ Health 2006;32(6): 493–501.

46. Irwin M, Clark C, Kennedy B, et al. Nocturnal catecholamines and immune function in insomniacs, depressed patients, and control subjects. Brain Behav Immun 2003;17(5):365–72.

47. Vgontzas AN, Chrousos GP. Sleep, the hypothalamic-pituitary-adrenal axis, and cytokines: multiple interactions and disturbances in sleep disorders. Endocrinol Metab Clin North Am 2002; 31(1):15–36.

48. Sephton SE, Lush E, Dedert EA, et al. Diurnal cortisol rhythm as a predictor of lung cancer survival. Brain Behav Immun 2013;30(SUPPL): S163–70.

49. Akıncı T, Melek Başar H. Relationship between sleep quality and the psychological status of patients hospitalised with COVID-19. Sleep Med 2021; 80(January):167–70.

50. Reiter RJ, Abreu-Gonzalez P, Marik PE, et al. Therapeutic Algorithm for use of melatonin in patients with COVID-19. Front Med (Lausanne) 2020;7:226.

51. Lange T, Dimitrov S, Born J. Effects of sleep and circadian rhythm on the human immune system: annals of the New York Academy of Sciences. Ann N Y Acad Sci 2010;1193:48–59.

52. Besedovsky L, Lange T, Haack M. The sleep-immune crosstalk in health and disease. Physiol Rev 2019;99(3):1325–80.

53. Teixeira KRC, dos Santos CP, de Medeiros LA, et al. Night workers have lower levels of antioxidant defenses and higher levels of oxidative stress damage when compared to day workers. Scientific Rep 2019;9(1):2021.

54. Maas MB, Kim M, Malkani RG, et al. Obstructive sleep apnea and risk of COVID-19 infection, hospitalization and respiratory failure. Sleep Breath 2020;25(2):1155–7.

55. Johnson KG, Sullivan SS, Nti A, et al. The impact of the COVID-19 pandemic on sleep medicine practices. J Clin Sleep Med 2021;17(1):79–87.

56. Iwu CJ, Iwu CD, Wiysonge CS. The occurrence of long COVID: a rapid review. Pan Afr Med J 2021; 38:65.

57. Chau SWH, Wong OWH, Ramakrishnan R, et al. History for some or lesson for all? A systematic review and meta-analysis on the immediate and long-term mental health impact of the 2002–2003 Severe Acute Respiratory Syndrome (SARS) outbreak. BMC Public Health 2021;21(1):670.

58. Benedict C, Cedernaes J. Could a good night's sleep improve COVID-19 vaccine efficacy? Lancet Respir Med 2021;9(5):447–8.

59. Kar A, Saxena K, Goyal A, et al. Assessment of obstructive sleep apnea in association with severity of COVID-19: a prospective observational study. Sleep Vigil 2021;5(1):111–8.

60. Lockhart SM, O'Rahilly S. When two pandemics meet: why is obesity associated with increased COVID-19 Mortality? Med (N Y) 2020;1(1):33–42.

61. force AC-t. Considerations for the practice of sleep medicine during COVID-19. Darian (Iran): American Academy of Sleep Medicine; 2021. Available at: https://aasm.org/covid-19-resources/considerations-practice-sleep-medicine/.

62. Gupta R, Kumar VM, Tripathi M, et al. Guidelines of the Indian society for sleep research (ISSR) for practice of sleep medicine during COVID-19. Sleep Vigil 2020;1–12.

63. Schiza S, Simonds A, Randerath W, et al. Sleep laboratories reopening and COVID-19: a European perspective. Eur Respir J 2021;57(3):2002722.

64. Crew EC, Baron KG, Grandner MA, et al. The society of behavioral sleep medicine (SBSM) COVID-19 task force: objectives and summary recommendations for managing sleep during a pandemic. Behav Sleep Med 2020;18(4):570–2.

65. Ayas NT, Fraser KL, Giannouli E, et al. Helping Canadian health care providers to optimize Sleep Disordered Breathing management for their patients during the COVID-19 pandemic. Can J Respir Crit Care Sleep Med 2020;4(2):81–2.

66. Insalaco G, Farra FD, Braghiroli A, et al. Sleep breathing disorders in the COVID-19 Era: Italian Thoracic Society Organizational Models for a correct approach to diagnosis and treatment. Respiration 2020;99(8):690–4.

67. Wilson KC, Kaminsky DA, Michaud G, et al. Restoring pulmonary and sleep services as the COVID-19 pandemic lessens. From an Association of Pulmonary, Critical Care, and Sleep Division Directors and American Thoracic Society-coordinated Task Force. Ann Am Thorac Soc 2020; 17(11):1343–51.

68. Stern M, Wagner MH, Thompson LA. Current and COVID-19 challenges with childhood and adolescent sleep. JAMA Pediatr 2020;174(11):1124.

69. Kelley GA, Kelley KS. Exercise and sleep: a systematic review of previous meta-analyses. J Evid Based Med 2017;10(1):26–36.

70. Rizzo D, Libman E, Baltzan M, et al. Impact of the COVID-19 pandemic on obstructive sleep apnea: recommendations for symptom management. J Clin Sleep Med 2021;17(3):429–34.

71. Riemann D, Baglioni C, Bassetti C, et al. European guideline for the diagnosis and treatment of insomnia. J Sleep Res 2017;26(6):675–700.

72. Sateia MJ, Buysse DJ, Krystal AD, et al. Clinical practice guideline for the pharmacologic treatment of chronic insomnia in adults: an American Academy of sleep medicine clinical practice guideline. J Clin Sleep Med 2017;13(2):307–49.

Sleep Complaints Among School Children

Ngan Yin Chan, PhD[a,1], Chun Ting Au, PhD[b,2], Shirley Xin Li, PhD, DClinPsy[c,d,3], Yun Kwok Wing, FRCPsych[a,1,*]

KEYWORDS

• Sleep complaints • Sleep disorders • Childhood sleep • Development

KEY POINTS

• Sleep complaints are common but often ignored and underrecognized in school childdren
• Sleep problems in school children are associated with a constellation of negative impact on children's development, learning, mental, and physical health
• Timely and appropriate management of pediatric sleep problems could alleviate the associated negative consequences
• Sleep problems are highly comorbid with neurodevelopmental disorders such as autism spectrum disorder (ASD) and attention deficit/hyperactive disorder (ADHD), and may exacerbate comorbid conditions and worsen the disease trajectory

INTRODUCTION

Adequate amount of quality sleep is particularly important for the optimal growth and health of children. However, up to 40% of children have sleep complaints including both night-time and daytime symptoms, such as trouble falling and maintaining sleep, snoring and unusual events during sleep (nightmare, sleepwalking), daytime sleepiness, and behavioral problems.[1] The presence of sleep problems not only lead to detrimental effects on children's health and well-being but also pose additional stress and burden on the caregivers and family. Nonetheless, sleep complaints in children are often overlooked and undertreated (**Table 1**).[2] Early identification and intervention are necessary to

mitigate and prevent negative consequences associated with sleep problems in school children.

NORMAL SLEEP IN CHILDREN

To define "abnormal" sleep in children, it is necessary to have a thorough understanding of "normal" sleep. It is well-established that sleep architecture and physiology change in parallel with physical growth and development. For example, there is abundant rapid eye movement (REM) sleep (50%) in infancy than in adults (20%), possibly due to its importance for early brain development.[3] Sleep is progressively consolidated into one single night of approximately 9 to 11 hours of sleep at the entry of primary school. Moreover, circadian

Conflict of interest: The other authors have indicated they have no conflict of interest.

[a] Li Chiu Kong Family Sleep Assessment Unit, Department of Psychiatry, Faculty of Medicine, The Chinese University of Hong Kong, Hong Kong SAR, China; [b] Department of Paediatrics, Faculty of Medicine, The Chinese University of Hong Kong, Hong Kong SAR, China; [c] Department of Psychology, The University of Hong Kong, Hong Kong SAR, China; [d] The State Key Laboratory of Brain and Cognitive Sciences, The University of Hong Kong, Hong Kong SAR, China

[1] 7/F, Li Chiu Kong Family Sleep Assessment Unit, Department of Psychiatry, Shatin Hospital, 33 A Kung Kok Street, Ma On Shan, Hong Kong, China

[2] 6/F, Lui Che Woo Clinical Sciences Building, Prince of Wales Hospital, 30-32 Ngan Shing Street, Shatin, Hong Kong, China

[3] C663, 6/F, The Jockey Club Tower Street, Pokfulam Road, Hong Kong Island, Hong Kong, China

* Corresponding author. 7/F, Department of Psychiatry, Shatin Hospital, 33 A Kung Kok Street, Ma On Shan, Hong Kong, China.

E-mail addresses: rachel.chan@cuhk.edu.hk (N.Y.C.); junau@cuhk.edu.hk (C.T.A.); shirleyx@hku.hk (S.X.L.); ykwing@cuhk.edu.hk (Y.K.W.)

Sleep Med Clin 17 (2022) 53–65
https://doi.org/10.1016/j.jsmc.2021.10.003
1556-407X/22/© 2021 Elsevier Inc. All rights reserved.

Table 1
Common sleep complaints and associated sleep problems in children

Common Sleep Complaints In Children		Common Sleep Problems in Children
Nighttime complaints	**Daytime complaints**	
Difficulty falling asleep	Excessive daytime Sleepiness	Sleep deprivation
Bedtime resistance	Difficulty in getting up in the morning	Insomnia
Difficulty maintaining sleep	Fatigue	Sleep-related breathing disorder
Night waking	Trouble concentrating	Disorders of arousal from NREM sleep
Snoring	Memory impairment	• Sleepwalking
Breathing pause during sleep	Hyperactivity	• Sleep terrors
Restless sleep	Impulsivity	REM-related parasomnia
	Morning headaches	• Nightmare disorder
	Mood disturbances or irritability	
	Low motivation	
	Lack of energy	

preference starts to emerge at school age with some children showing an increased preference for relatively late bedtime.[4] A combination of both biological factors and external factors such as early school start time and environmental constraints determine the sleep-wake pattern in school children.[5,6]

SLEEP DEPRIVATION
Associated sleep complaints

Nighttime: late bedtime
   Daytime: difficulty in getting up in the morning, excessive daytime sleepiness, fatigue, trouble concentrating, cognitive impairment, hyperactivity, impulsivity, and morning headaches.

Epidemiology

Recent evidence showed that sleep deprivation among children is an emerging pandemic across the world, affecting 25% to 40% of normally developing children.[7] The average sleep duration during school days is approximately 8 hours per night for school children.[7] In other words, a substantial proportion of school children is sleeping with a duration of sleep at the range of late adolescents and adults. Such "adult pattern" of childhood sleep duration is worrisome as early sleep habits tend to persist with age.[2] There is also empirical evidence suggesting a secular trend of reduced sleep duration in children across different regions.[7,8] For example, a secular trend of decreasing sleep time from early 2000s to early 2010s was observed in Hong Kong children who were also sleeping about 40 minutes less than Shanghai children.[8]

Impact

The manifestations of sleepiness in children are conspicuously different from adults. For example, children tend to respond to sleep deprivation by externalizing their behaviors, such as increased irritability, hyperactivity, and inattention.[9] In addition, the curtailment of sleep impairs children's cognitive performance and learning capacity and has been identified as a risk factor for obesity, hyperlipidemia, hypertension, and emotional problems.[9]

Management

Sleep education is one of the potential interventions to improve children's sleep habits. In particular, the healthy attitude and correct beliefs about the sleep of most parents and children are inadequate.[10] Thus, psychoeducation is important, especially with the active involvement of school and parents, who play a vital and active role in cultivating children's sleep habits. It is important to prioritize sleep and establish good sleep habits starting at a young age. Nonetheless, sleep education may be able to enhance sleep knowledge, but it may not be able to lead to the behavioral translation into longer sleep duration.[10]

INSOMNIA
Associated sleep complaints

Nighttime: difficulty falling asleep, difficulty maintaining sleep, bedtime resistance, and night waking.
   Daytime: difficulty in getting up in the morning, excessive daytime sleepiness, fatigue, trouble concentrating, cognitive impairment, hyperactivity, impulsivity, morning headaches, and mood disturbance.

Epidemiology

The estimated prevalence of childhood insomnia symptoms ranges from 20% to 30% depending on the diagnostic criteria.[11] When more stringent operational criteria are applied, the estimated prevalence was 4% to 7% in the prepubertal children (**Box 1**).[12] There is a surge of the prevalence of insomnia in late pubertal stage with female predominance, affecting 12.2% in girls and 9.1% in boys.[12] Previous research also supported that childhood insomnia, if left untreated, may persist over time (eg, 15% over 5-year follow-up), albeit the persistence rate may be lower than that of the adolescent and adult insomnia.[13]

Pathophysiology

The causes of childhood insomnia may be related to a complex interaction of biological, circadian, neurodevelopmental, behavioral, and environmental factors. In particular, a strong familial aggregation and the genetic underpinning of insomnia has been reported.[13–15] Those children with a parent who has insomnia are at 2 to 3 times increased risk of having insomnia than their counterparts.[13–15] The interaction of predisposing factors and a wide range of external factors, such as poor sleep hygiene, excessive media use, and school burden may increase the risk of insomnia in children. Furthermore, several medical and psychiatric conditions including depression, anxiety, and neurodevelopmental disorders (NDDs) may also contribute to the occurrence of childhood insomnia.

Impact

Various cross-sectional and longitudinal studies emphasized the association of childhood insomnia with emotional disturbances, externalizing behavioral problems, cognitive impairment, suicidality, and family disruption.[16,17] For example, prefrontal cortical dysfunction is evidenced in children with insomnia, which could lead to impairment in executive function with further negative impact on working memory, emotional regulation, and attention.[18] Moreover, insomnia is associated with elevated risk of future psychopathology including depression, anxiety, and suicidality.[17] Importantly, the resolution of insomnia might relieve these symptoms, suggesting the importance of addressing sleep problems in children and adolescents.

Treatment

For young children, behavioral interventions are often recommended as the first-line treatment of managing childhood insomnia. Examples of these main therapeutic components include graduated extinction, scheduled awakenings, and bedtime routine.[19]

For older children, cognitive behavioral therapy for insomnia (CBT-I) targeting maladaptive behaviors and cognition has received increasing evidence.[16] The available findings consistently supported the positive effects of CBT-I including reducing sleep onset latency, increasing sleep efficiency, reducing problematic sleep association, as well as anxiety.[20] It is of note that the positive gains were maintained at 12-month follow-up.[20]

For pharmacologic treatment, there is currently no medication approved by the US Food and Drug Administration (FDA) in treating childhood insomnia. In a national survey, approximately 90% of child psychiatrists in the United States recommended over the counter medication for managing insomnia in children and adolescents, with melatonin being the most frequently dispensed drug.[21,22] Due to the concern about the safety and clinical efficacy of medication usage in the pediatric population, pharmacotherapy should be used as a supplementary to behavioral intervention,[23] and the prescription should be carefully selected based on the clinician's best judgment in accordance with the patient's presenting complaints, disease severity, and comorbidities.

SLEEP-RELATED BREATHING DISORDER
Associated sleep complaints

Nighttime: night waking and sweating, restless sleep, snoring, and breathing pause during sleep.

Daytime: excessive daytime sleepiness, trouble concentrating, cognitive impairment, hyperactivity, impulsivity, morning headaches, and mood disturbance.

Box 1
Insomnia

Clinical manifestation:

1. Inability to fall asleep,

2. Bedtime resistance,

3. Difficulty to stay asleep

4. Waking earlier than the desired wakeup time,

The problems exist even when the child has sufficient opportunity and appropriate environment to sleep

Chronic insomnia: at least three times a week for at least 3 months

Short term insomnia: at least three times a week, less than 3 months

Prevalence: 4% to 7% for chronic insomnia; 20% to 30% for insomnia symptoms

Sleep-related breathing disorder (SRBD) encompass a wide spectrum ranging from primary snoring to obstructive sleep apnea syndrome (OSAS).[24] Primary snoring is defined as snoring without abnormal ventilation, while OSAS is characterized by partial or complete upper airway obstruction despite respiratory effort, which disturbs sleep and ventilation during sleep.[24] The clinical presentations of children with OSAS often include habitual and loud snoring, mouth breathing, choking, abnormal sleeping position, and restless sleep (**Box 2**).[24,25]

Epidemiology

For habitual snoring, the estimated prevalence ranged from 2% to 35%,[26,27] whereas for OSAS as confirmed by polysomnography, the prevalence is about 1%–5% in the childhood population.[25,28,29] In particular, childhood obesity has been considered as one of the major risk factors to OSAS, affecting about 50% of obese children.[30,31] The highest incidence of childhood OSAS is at 3–6 years old, possibly because children at this period have the largest tonsils and adenoids.[32] In addition, boys are more likely to have OSAS than girls.[25,33] This is in parallel with the evidence showing that girls are more likely to have a complete resolution of OSA during the transition to adolescence.[34,35]

Pathophysiology

The pathophysiology of OSAS is multifactorial including both anatomic obstruction and neuromotor factors.[36] With the increasing prevalence of childhood obesity, obesity is now recognized as a major factor predisposing to the development of OSAS in children.[37] Interestingly, the heritability of obstructive apnea–hypopnea index (OAHI) was

only present in overweight children,[38] suggesting that obesity-related OSAS is a distinct subtype in children.

In general, children with OSAS often have enlarged tonsils and adenoids, suggesting the primary role of these anatomic structures in the pathogenesis of OSAS. More recently, some new anatomic markers, including lower hyoid bone position (a potential marker of tongue enlargement) and lateral parapharyngeal wall thickness have been shown to correlate with childhood OSAS independent of obesity and tonsil size.[39] Moreover, the presence of craniofacial abnormalities such as cleft palate, micrognathia, and midface hypoplasia could further pose additional risk of OSAS.[36]

However, not all children with these anatomic deficits will develop OSAS, and for children who have undergone adenotonsillectomy (AT), OSAS could redevelop in their adolescence, suggesting that other factors such as alterations in upper airway muscle responsiveness and central ventilatory drive might play critical roles in the development of childhood OSAS.[36]

Impact

Untreated and chronic OSAS pose a significant risk to children's development and health. The most reported impairments are neurobehavioral and neurocognitive deficits. For example, behavioral problems including inattention, hyperactivity, aggression, and disruptive behaviors are commonly found.[40] Although multiple neurocognitive dysfunctions such as executive function and vigilance are suggested to occur in children with OSAS, there are inconsistencies in the literature, possibly related to the methodological variations and limitations of the studies.[41] Interestingly, several randomized controlled studies reported that AT did not improve objectively assessed cognitive function including executive function,[42] learning and memory,[43] intellectual ability,[44] and attention.[45] Nonetheless, parent-reported behaviors[42] and quality of life[45] were significantly improved following AT.

Cardiovascular and metabolic disturbances are commonly observed among children with OSAS.[41,46] Elevated blood pressure, a well-established risk factor for cardiovascular problems across all age groups, has been demonstrated to be associated with childhood OSAS. Longitudinal studies have found that childhood OSA is associated with elevated BP at 4-year follow-up and through adulthood.[35,46]

Treatment

AT is the first-line treatment of childhood OSAS, especially for moderate-to-severe OSAS (AHI > 5)

Box 2
Obstructive sleep apnea

Clinical manifestations:

- Habitual and loud snoring
- Mouth breathing, choking
- Prone sleeping position
- Restless sleep
- Bedwetting, night sweating

Prevalence: 1% to 5% in pediatric population

Pathophysiology:

- Adenotonsillar hypertrophy
- Obesity
- Allergic rhinitis

in nonobese children. However, for mild OSAS (AHI between 1 and 5), there is no established consensus on the intervention.[47] Constant monitoring with supportive care might be an appropriate option for mild and normal weight cases.[48,49] Although AT can effectively reduce AHI, residual OSA after AT is an important and common issue. A multicentre retrospective study found that OSA severity reduced significantly after AT, but only 27% of them had complete resolution.[50] Particularly, obese and older children are less likely to benefit from surgical treatment and are at increased risk for persistent OSA.[37] On top of that, randomized controlled trials consistently demonstrated significant weight gain after adentonsillectomy in school-aged children.[45,50] Thus, risk–benefit ratio has to be evaluated carefully especially for children with mild OSAS.[37]

Alternative nonsurgical interventions for children without adenotonsillar hypertrophy or those with residual OSA after AT may also be beneficial to those with mild disease. Such interventions include weight loss, positive airway pressure (PAP) therapy, oral appliances, myofunctional therapy, and medication such as nasal steroids.[51] PAP receives strong and empirical evidence in reducing OSA symptoms in children with different severity.[49]

PARASOMNIAS

Parasomnias are common in children. Three main types of parasomnias are classified based on the International Classification Of Sleep Disorders, 3rd edition (ICSD-3) including (1) disorders of arousal from non-REM sleep, (2) parasomnias usually associated with REM sleep, and (3) other parasomnias[52] (**Table 2**). Most of the parasomnias often decrease with age and are considered self-limiting and benign in children. The major clinical manifestations of parasomnias include abnormal movements, emotional arousal, and autonomic activity which are thought to be associated with CNS activation.

Disorders of Arousal from Non-Rapid Eye Movement Sleep

Associated Sleep Complaints

Nighttime: night terror and automatism in NREM parasomnia, night waking, abnormal movement, partial arousal, comorbid symptoms of OSA, and RLS.

Daytime: daytime sleepiness, fatigue, and emotional disturbance.

The disorder of arousal parasomnia includes sleep terror, sleepwalking, and confusional arousals. It often occurs in the first part of the night which constitutes abundant slow wave sleep. The apparent "dissociation" between sleep and awakening leads to autonomic activation, confusion, and disturbed perception. Confusional arousals are more frequently present in children who are younger than 5 years old, whereas sleepwalking and sleep terrors are more common in school-aged children.[53–56]

Sleepwalking

Sleepwalking is also known as somnambulism and is characterized by partial arousal during slow

Table 2
Comparison between common parasomnias in school children

	NREM Parasomnias		REM Parasomnia
	Sleepwalking	**Sleep Terror**	**Nightmares**
Age of peak onset (y)	10	4–6	6–10
Prevalence	5%[53]	1%–6%[54]	5%[55]
Clinical manifestation	Partial arousal, accompanied with either clam or agitated behaviors with a wide range of complexity and duration	Partial arousal, extreme fears, and panic and associated with marked automatic nervous system activation suddenly sit upright, or even jump out of bed during the episode	Accompany with intense feelings of fear and terror and dreamers can recall the details of the dream content
Time of occurrence	SWS	SWS	REM
Duration of the episode	2–30 min	1–10 min	3–20 min

Abbreviations: REM, rapid eye movement; SWS, slow wave sleep.

wave sleep, accompanied by a wide range of behavioral complexity and varying duration. Sleepwalkers can perform complex automatic behaviors such as walking without response to the environmental stimuli.[57,58] Most sleepwalking episodes are harmless, but in some cases, sleepwalking could result in injury to patients themselves or to others.[59] The estimated lifetime prevalence is 6.9% according to a systematic review with more than 100,000 subjects.[53] The 12-month prevalence is significantly higher in children (5.0%) than in adults (1.5%). The peak prevalence of sleepwalking is observed at age 10 (13.4%) with no apparent gender difference.[53]

Sleep terror

Sleep terror is also known as night terrors or pavor nocturnus. Similar to sleepwalking, it consists of partial arousal from slow wave sleep and is characterized by extreme fears and panic, marked autonomic activation including mydriasis, sweating, screaming, shouting, or crying behaviors.[60] The child may suddenly sit upright, or even jump out of bed during the episode, yet the speech and motor function are somewhat disorganized, and confused. The episode often lasts from a few minutes to 30 minutes before the child returns to sleep. The estimated prevalence rate is ranging from 1% to 6% and is more commonly reported in children with a peak of prevalence during 4 to 6 years old.[54,61] The lifetime prevalence is approximately 10% with male predominance in the pediatric population.[56] It has been shown that childhood sleep terror is a risk factor for sleepwalking with one-third of children who had early experiences of sleep terrors was found to develop sleepwalking in later ages.[2,56]

Etiology

Albeit that the exact etiology of NREM parasomnias is unknown, factors that contribute to the arousal from slow wave sleep might increase the occurrence of NREM parasomnia. These include developmental, genetic, psychosocial, and environmental factors.[57,58]

There is clear evidence that both sleepwalking and sleep terrors are heritable with a strong genetic predisposition.[62] For example, approximately half of children who report sleepwalking had a positive parental history of sleepwalking.[56] Similarly, children whose parents have sleep terrors are 10 times more likely to have sleep terrors than those without positive family history.[62] In addition, human leukocyte antigen (HLA) DQB1*04 and DQB1*05:01 alleles are commonly presented in children with NREM parasomnia.[63,64]

Given that NREM parasomnia rarely occurs after puberty, developmental factors such as neurodevelopmental immaturity and changes in sleep architecture might potentially lead to the onset.[57,58] It has been hypothesized that cortical GABAergic inhibition and cholinergic inhibitory circuits are "less efficient" and immature to inhibit movement during slow wave sleep during childhood.[65] This is in accordance with the disappearance of parasomnia during adolescence and adulthood.[61]

Children with genetic susceptibility do not always develop arousal disorders unless there is presence of priming factors. Priming factors are referred to those intrinsic or environmental factors that affect slow wave sleep instability which eventually triggers or precipitates the episode of NREM parasomnia.[66] For example, factors that deepen slow wave sleep, such as prolonged sleep deprivation or irregular sleep wake pattern, have been shown to be associated with more frequent and severe sleepwalking episodes.[59,66,67] Other factors that are associated with sleep fragmentation and arousal might also trigger the onset of NREM parasomnia. These include fever (>38.3C),[68] stress and anxiety,[69] comorbid sleep disorders (especially OSAS, restless legs syndrome),[70,71] chronic pain, and environmental stimuli (noisy or stimulating sleep environment).[72]

Impact

Arousal disorders in children are generally considered benign, particularly if they occur occasionally. However, chronic and recurrent arousal disorders could pose additional risk to both children and their families.[60,63] For example, more frequent and severe episodes of sleepwalking or sleep terrors may lead to sleep disruption, self-initiated injuries, property damage, and involuntary aggression to others. In addition, these unusual sleep events may cause significant parental distress and anxiety.[57,61] Children presented with recurrent arousal disorders also have a higher risk for daytime impairment, behavioral, and emotional problems.

Management

The treatment approach mainly lies in the identification and elimination of priming factors, environmental modifications as well as providing parental reassurance.[1,57] For those with recurrent attacks, further sleep investigations to rule out comorbid and highly treatable sleep disorders such as OSAS may be needed. In addition, parental education is needed to promote good sleep hygiene practice to avoid sleep deprivation and adopt appropriate environmental protective measures to prevent and minimize potential injuries during the episode. A behavioral treatment with scheduled awakening is suggested for children who have a predictable time of arousal behaviors. Quietly waking children half an hour before their usual time for the parasomnia episode may abort the undesirable event.

For pharmacologic approach, there is some clinical evidence for the efficacy of benzodiazepines (eg, clonazepam) and tricyclic antidepressants in treating arousal disorders in children, yet the medications should be started with low-dose and close monitoring due to the potential side effects such as daytime sedation.[57,60] However, randomized controlled trials are needed to further evaluate the clinical efficacy of the pharmacologic approach in treating arousal disorders in children.

RAPID EYE MOVEMENT-RELATED PARASOMNIA
Nightmare disorder

Associated sleep complaints
Nighttime: night waking, dreams with frightening content, sleep-related anxiety, intense feelings of fear, and terror following night waking.

Daytime: daytime sleepiness and anxiety.

Nightmares are disturbing mental experiences that result in awakening from sleep. It is defined as "an internally generated conscious experience or dream sequence that seems vivid and real" (ICSD-3).[52] In young children, monsters or fantastical imagery represent the main characteristic of nightmare content. The frightening content of the dreams often awakes the children, making them not be able to return to sleep.

Epidemiology
Up to 75% of children occasionally report nightmare,[73] whereas a frequent nightmare (at least once per week) affects 5% to 20% of children with the peak onset at 6–10 years of age[55,74,75] Boys and girls are equally affected by nightmare in school children with female preponderance emerging in young adolescents.[76,77] Albeit most of the nightmares can resolve as children age, about 30% of the children have persistent nightmare.[78]

Pathophysiology
Dreaming is thought to be a process for memory consolidation, and for enabling fear extinction.[79,80] In contrast, nightmare is a process that reinforce fear experience by activating amygdala during REM sleep, which is postulated to be an important component in the pathogenesis of nightmares.[81,82] In addition, hyperarousal, a central component in insomnia and posttraumatic stress disorder might be implicated in nightmare disorder due to their high coexistence.[80] It is possible that the enhanced arousal interacts with impaired fear extinction, in the presence of precipitating traumatic events or stressors, results in a nightmare experience.

Impact
Children who have frequent nightmare (at least once per week) are more likely to have comorbid sleep problems including insomnia and parasomnia. Nightmares in children have found to be independently associated with emotional and behavioral difficulties.[55] The presence of nightmare has been reported as a risk factor for childhood psychopathology.[55,73] Mindell and Barrett found that elementary-aged children who experience nightmare tend to be more anxious than their peers without night disturbances.[73] In older children, frequent nightmares are found to be associated with the risk for suicidality and possibly psychotic experience.[83,84]

Treatment
Occasional nightmare is common in children. Parents should reassure their children that the occurrence of occasional bad dream is normal because the frequency and intensity of the episodes will progressively resolve with age. Behavioral suggestions are recommended, including limiting the children's exposure to precipitating factors of nightmare such as violent content or emotional arousals few hours before bedtime.[85] Identification and management of daytime stressors are also recommended to reduce the nightmare episodes. If the occurrence of nightmare is associated with other mental disorders such as anxiety or PTSD, appropriate intervention may be needed.[85] Imagery rehearsal therapy (IRT) and CBT are the most frequently studied psychological treatment of nightmare in adults.[86,87] However, the research on the clinical efficacy of these treatment approaches in school children is lacking and conflicting.[87,88]

RESTLESS LEGS SYNDROME
Associated sleep complaints

Nighttime: trouble falling asleep, difficulty maintaining sleep, night waking, intense urge to move the leg, and unpleasant leg sensations.

Daytime: intense urge to move the leg, unpleasant leg sensations, and daytime sleepiness.

To diagnose childhood RLS, a consensus published in 2003 and further updated in 2013 outlined that in addition to the essential 'adult' RLS criteria, there is also a need for age-specific vocabulary used by children in describing their own discomfort sensations and the associated impairment might be more apparent in behavioral and learning aspects in children (**Box 3**).[89,90]

Epidemiology

RLS affects 2% to 4% of children and increases to 17% in general pediatric clinics.[91–93] For example, Picchietti and colleagues (2007) estimated that 1.9% of children aged between 8- to 11-years-old children had RLS with large proportion of them experience moderate to severe RLS symptoms ($\geq$2 times per week).[90] Approximately 30% of adults who suffered from RLS recalled the early symptoms before the age of 10 years.[94] Gender difference of RLS emerged in late adolescents with female preponderance.[95]

Pathophysiology

Multiple factors have been identified to play key roles in RLS such as genetic predisposition, dopamine dysfunction, and iron deficiency. Strong familial aggregation and several genetic variants such as PTPRD, BTBD9, and MEIS1 genes are associated with RLS.[96,97] Another contributor to RLS is inadequate dopamine production and blockade.[97] As iron plays a key role in the synthesis of dopamine, emerging evidence suggests that children with RLS have low ferritin and iron deficiency.[98]

Impact

Increase evidence suggests a constellation of adverse effects of RLS in sleep, emotion, behavior, cognitive, and health in children. A recent systematic review provides empirical evidence that RLS in children is comorbid with several somatic and neuropsychiatric symptoms.[91,99] This might also partly explain the close connection between RLS and attention-deficit/hyperactivity disorder (ADHD). Inattention, hyperactivity, and restlessness following sleep disruption might mimic ADHD symptoms in children with RLS.[93] In addition, somatic symptoms such as migraine and growing pains are increasingly recognized in pediatric RLS, and the presence of these complaints are associated with increased severity of RLS.[99]

Treatment

For nonpharmacological approach, identification of potential factors that aggravate RLS symptoms is recommended as the initial step. Several medications (eg, selective serotonin reuptake inhibitor, metoclopramide, and diphenhydramine) and poor lifestyle practice have been reported to increase RLS.[100,101] Removal of these precipitating factors might alleviate RLS. Parents are encouraged to promote good sleep hygiene practice in children such as limiting caffeinated consumption, avoiding sleep deprivation, and maintaining a regular sleep schedule for managing RLS.

There is currently no medication approved by the US FDA for managing pediatric RLS. The dopaminergic medications including levodopa, ropinirole, and pramipexole, and other medications such as $\alpha2\delta$ ligands (pregabalin and gabapentin) are possibly effective in alleviating RLS in the childhood population.[102] Moreover, children with RLS presented with iron deficiency and low iron stores may benefit from iron therapy, but recent guideline addresses the necessity of more empirical evidence in the clinical efficacy of iron treatment of pediatric RLS.[103]

CROSS-CULTURAL DIFFERENCES IN SLEEP PROBLEMS

Cultural factors are important determinants of sleep practice and behaviors in children.[104] Although many sleep problems are universal across cultures, the uniqueness of each culture still partially defines parent's and child's behaviors. The culturally embedded behaviors include cosleeping, bedtime routines, sleep environment, and napping behaviors.[104] For example, cosleeping is generally encouraged and accepted in Asian countries including China, Korea, and Japan with approximately 60% of children bed-sharing with their parents, which is much higher than their American counterparts (15%).[105] These culturally determined behaviors might be the possible

---

Box 3
Restless legs syndrome/Willis–Ekbom disease

Clinical manifestations:

- Intense and irresistible urges to move the legs due to the unpleasant and discomfort sensations

- Increased discomfort feeling in the evening

- Rest or inactivity could exacerbate the discomfort. Movement could partially relieve the uncomfortable sensations.

Prevalence: 2% to 4% in pediatric population

Pathophysiology:

- Genetic predisposition and susceptibility

- Inadequate dopamine production and blockade

- Iron deficiency

reasons leading to the differences in severity and frequency of sleep problems observed between Asian and Western countries.[106] For example, Asian children and adolescents consistently report later bedtime and shorter sleep duration than their European counterparts.[7] Even within the same country, sleep patterns are different among children in Hong Kong and Shanghai.[8] The exact reason for such subcultural variations remains unclear, but this observation suggested the importance of cultural considerations in clinical assessment of pediatric sleep problems.[5]

SLEEP PROBLEMS IN CHILDREN WITH SPECIAL NEEDS

A markedly higher prevalence (40%–80%) of sleep problems are observed in children with NDDs such as autism spectrum disorder (ASD), ADHD, and intellectual disability.[107–109] The occurrence of sleep problems often exacerbates the comorbid conditions and worsen the disease trajectory. Increasing evidence has suggested that it is essential to provide sleep treatment in children with NDDs to ameliorate associated negative impact including daytime impairment, cognitive deficits, and family distress. A recent review has supported the clinical efficacy of both nonpharmacological and pharmacologic treatment of insomnia in children with NDDs,[110] even though the evidence was limited by the heterogeneity of the studies, small sample size, and lack of robust randomized controlled design.[111]

SUMMARY

Sleep problems are prevalent in school children. Although some of the sleep problems may be benign in nature with spontaneous resolution with increasing age, a proportion of them may persist into adolescence and adulthood, leading to significant distress and repercussion to both children and their families. Timely sleep intervention is essential to ameliorate the negative consequences. It is necessary for parents and children to acquire adequate sleep knowledge and to maintain good sleep habits thereby reducing the development of sleep problems in children.

CLINICS CARE POINTS

- Detailed and comprehensive assessment on medical, developmental as well as family history is essential when diagnosing pediatric sleep disorders.

- It is important to explore the underlying co-morbid physical and mental conditions as they could potentially complicate the sleep problems, and have implications for selecting the respective treatment approach.

- Parental involvement is necessary to collect necessary information for making the clinical diagnosis, particularly in young children.

- Screening and assessment tools such as sleep diary, self-reported or parent-reported sleep questionnaire are useful for supporting the diagnosis, whereas a comprehensive objective sleep assessment, such as polysomnography, is considered necessary if the child is suspected of having OSA.

- Behavioral intervention such as sleep hygiene and parental education should always be considered as the initial treatment approach.

- Medications should only be prescribed when behavioral intervention fails. Close monitoring and regular assessment of the potential side effects are highly encouraged when providing pharmacotherapy.

DISCLOSURE

Y.K. Wing reports grants from Research Grant Council of University Grants Committee, Health and Medical Research Fund, Hong Kong SAR; received personal fees for delivering a lecture from Eisai and sponsorship from Lundbeck HK Limited.

REFERENCE

1. Thiedke CC. Sleep disorders and sleep problems in childhood. Am Fam Physician 2001;63:277–84.
2. Gregory AM, O'Connor TG. Sleep problems in childhood: a longitudinal study of developmental change and association with behavioral problems. J Am Acad Child Adolesc Psychiatry 2002;41:964–71.
3. El Shakankiry HM. Sleep physiology and sleep disorders in childhood. Nat Sci Sleep 2011;3:101–14.
4. Abbott A. Physiology: an end to adolescence. Nature 2005;433:27.
5. Jenni OG, O'Connor BB. Children's sleep: an interplay between culture and biology. Pediatrics 2005; 115:204–16.
6. Zhang JH, Li AM, Fok TF, et al. Roles of parental sleep/wake patterns, socioeconomic status, and daytime activities in the sleep/wake patterns of children. U105. J Pediatr-us 2010;156:606.
7. Matricciani L, Olds T, Petkov J. In search of lost sleep: secular trends in the sleep time of school-aged children and adolescents. Sleep Med Rev 2012;16:203–11.

8. Wang GH, Zhang JH, Lam SP, et al. Ten-year secular trends in sleep/wake patterns in Shanghai and Hong Kong school-aged children: a Tale of two Cities. J Clin Sleep Med 2019;15:1495–502.

9. Orzel-Gryglewska J. Consequences of sleep deprivation. Int J Occup Med Env 2010;23:95–114.

10. Wing YK, Chan NY, Yu MWM, et al. A school-based sleep education program for adolescents: a cluster randomized trial. Pediatrics 2015;135:E635–43.

11. Fricke-Oerkermann L, Pluck J, Schredl M, et al. Prevalence and course of sleep problems in childhood. Sleep 2007;30:1371–7.

12. Zhang J, Chan NY, Lam SP, et al. Emergence of sex differences in insomnia symptoms in adolescents: a large-Scale school-based study. Sleep 2016;39:1563–70.

13. Zhang J, Lam SP, Li SX, et al. Longitudinal course and outcome of chronic insomnia in Hong Kong Chinese children: a 5-year follow-up study of a community-based cohort. Sleep 2011;34:1395–402.

14. Zhang J, Lam SP, Li SX, et al. Insomnia, sleep quality, pain, and somatic symptoms: sex differences and shared genetic components. Pain 2012;153:666–73.

15. Lane JM, Jones SE, Dashti HS, et al. Biological and clinical insights from genetics of insomnia symptoms. Nat Genet 2019;51:387–93.

16. Nunes ML, Bruni O. Insomnia in childhood and adolescence: clinical aspects, diagnosis, and therapeutic approach. J Pediat-brazil 2015;91:S26–35.

17. Fortier-Brochu E, Beaulieu-Bonneau S, Ivers H, et al. Insomnia and daytime cognitive performance: a meta-analysis. Sleep Med Rev 2012;16:83–94.

18. Bos SC, Gomes A, Clemente V, et al. Sleep and behavioral/emotional problems in children: a population-based study. Sleep Med 2009;10:66–74.

19. Owens J. Insomnia in children and adolescents. J Clin Sleep Med 2005;1:E454–8.

20. Schlarb AA, Bihlmaier I, Velten-Schurian K, et al. Short- and long-term effects of CBT-I in groups for school-age children suffering from chronic insomnia: the KiSS-Program. Behav Sleep Med 2018;16:380–97.

21. Hartz I, Furu K, Bratlid T, et al. Hypnotic drug use among 0-17 year olds during 2004-2011: a nationwide prescription database study. Scand J Public Healt 2012;40:704–11.

22. Owens JA, Rosen CL, Mindell JA, et al. Use of pharmacotherapy for insomnia in child psychiatry practice: a national survey. Sleep Med 2010;11:692–700.

23. Ekambaram V, Owens J. Medications used for pediatric insomnia. Child Adol Psych Cl 2021;30:85–99.

24. Li AM, Au CT, So HK, et al. Prevalence and risk factors of habitual snoring in primary school children. Chest 2010;138:519–27.

25. Li AM, So HK, Au CT, et al. Epidemiology of obstructive sleep apnoea syndrome in Chinese children: a two-phase community study. Thorax 2010;65:991–7.

26. Dehlink E, Tan HL. Update on paediatric obstructive sleep apnoea. J Thorac Dis 2016;8:224–35.

27. DelRosso LM. Epidemiology and diagnosis of pediatric obstructive sleep apnea. Curr Prob Pediatr Ad 2016;46:2–6.

28. Rosen CL, Larkin EK, Kirchner HL, et al. Prevalence and risk factors for sleep-disordered breathing in 8-to 11-year-old children: association with race and prematurity. J Pediatr-us 2003;142:383–9.

29. Bixler EO, Vgontzas AN, Lin HM, et al. Sleep disordered breathing in children in a general population sample: prevalence and risk factors. Sleep 2009;32:731–6.

30. Kalra M, Inge T, Garcia V, et al. Obstructive sleep apnea in extremely overweight adolescents undergoing bariatric surgery. Obes Res 2005;13:1175–9.

31. Marcus CL, Curtis S, Koerner CB, et al. Evaluation of pulmonary function and polysomnography in obese children and adolescents. Pediatr Pulm 1996;21:176–83.

32. Wing YK, Hui SH, Pak WM, et al. A controlled study of sleep related disordered breathing in obese children. Arch Dis Child 2003;88:1043–7.

33. Inoshita A, Kasai T, Matsuoka R, et al. Age-stratified sex differences in polysomnographic findings and pharyngeal morphology among children with obstructive sleep apnea. J Thorac Dis 2018;10:6702–10.

34. Chan KC, Au CT, Hui LL, et al. How OSA evolves from childhood to young adulthood natural history from a 10-year follow-up study. Chest 2019;156:120–30.

35. Chan KCC, Au CT, Hui LL, et al. Childhood OSA an independent determinant of blood pressure in adulthood: longitudinal follow-up study. Thorax 2020;75:422–31.

36. Marcus CL. Pathophysiology of childhood obstructive sleep apnea: current concepts. Resp Physiol 2000;119:143–54.

37. Au CT, Li AM. Obstructive sleep breathing disorders. Pediatr Clin N Am 2009;56:243.

38. Au CT, Zhang JH, Cheung JYF, et al. Familial aggregation and heritability of obstructive sleep apnea using children Probands. J Clin Sleep Med 2019;15:1561–70.

39. Au CT, Chan KCC, Liu KH, et al. Potential anatomic markers of obstructive sleep apnea in Prepubertal children. J Clin Sleep Med 2018;14:1979–86.

40. Chervin RD, Archbold KH, Dillon JE, et al. Inattention, hyperactivity, and symptoms of sleep-disordered breathing. Pediatrics 2002;109:449–56.

41. Muzumdar H, Arens R. Physiological effects of obstructive sleep apnea syndrome in childhood. Respir Physiol Neurobiol 2013;188:370–82.

42. Marcus CL, Moore RH, Rosen CL, et al. A randomized trial of adenotonsillectomy for childhood sleep apnea. New Engl J Med 2013;368:2366–76.

43. Taylor HG, Bowen SR, Beebe DW, et al. Cognitive effects of adenotonsillectomy for obstructive sleep apnea. Pediatrics 2016;138(2):e20154458.

44. Waters K, Chawla J, Harris MA, et al. Cognition after early tonsillectomy for mild OSA. Pediatrics 2020;145(2):e20191450.

45. Au CT, Chan KCC, Lee DLY, et al. Effect of surgical intervention for mild childhood obstructive sleep apnoea on attention and behavioural outcomes: a randomized controlled study. Respirology 2021;26(7):690–9.

46. Li AM, Au CT, Ng C, et al. A 4-year prospective follow-up study of childhood OSA and its association with BP. Chest 2014;145:1255–63.

47. Gozal D, Tan HL, Kheirandish-Gozal L. Treatment of obstructive sleep apnea in children: handling the unknown with precision. J Clin Med 2020;9(3):888.

48. Farber JM. Clinical practice guideline: diagnosis and management of childhood obstructive sleep apnea syndrome. Pediatrics 2002;110:1255–7. author reply -7.

49. Marcus CL, Brooks LJ, Draper KA, et al. Diagnosis and management of childhood obstructive sleep apnea syndrome. Pediatrics 2012;130:e714–55.

50. Bhattacharjee R, Kheirandish-Gozal L, Spruyt K, et al. Adenotonsillectomy outcomes in treatment of obstructive sleep apnea in children A multicenter retrospective study. Am J Resp Crit Care 2010;182:676–83.

51. Chan CCK, Au CT, Lam HS, et al. Intranasal corticosteroids for mild childhood obstructive sleep apnea - a randomized, placebo-controlled study. Sleep Med 2015;16:358–63.

52. Sateia MJ. International classification of sleep disorders-third edition: highlights and modifications. Chest 2014;146:1387–94.

53. Stallman HM, Kohler M. Prevalence of sleepwalking: a systematic review and meta-analysis. Plos One 2016;11(11):e0164769.

54. Medicine AAoS. International classification of sleep disorders. In: Diagnostic and coding manual. 2nd edition. Westchester, Illinois: American Academy of Sleep Medicine; 2005.

55. Li SX, Yu MWM, Lam SP, et al. Frequent nightmares in children: familial aggregation and associations with parent-reported behavioral and mood problems. Sleep 2011;34:487–93.

56. Petit D, Pennestri MH, Paquet J, et al. Childhood sleepwalking and sleep terrors a longitudinal study of prevalence and familial aggregation. Jama Pediatr 2015;169:653–8.

57. Mason TBA, Pack AI. Pediatric parasomnias. Sleep 2007;30:141–51.

58. Howell MJ. Parasomnias: an updated review. Neurotherapeutics 2012;9:753–75.

59. Rauch PK, Stern TA. Life-threatening injuries resulting from sleepwalking and night terrors. Psychosomatics 1986;27:62–4.

60. Leung AKC, Leung AAM, Wong AHC, et al. Sleep terrors: an updated review. Curr Pediatr Rev 2020;16:176–82.

61. Avidan AY, Kaplish N. The parasomnias: epidemiology, clinical features, and diagnostic approach. Clin Chest Med 2010;31:353.

62. Kales A, Soldatos CR, Bixler EO, et al. Hereditary factors in sleepwalking and night terrors. Br J Psychiat 1980;137:111–8.

63. Irfan M, Schenck CH, Howell MJ. Non-rapid eye movement sleep and overlap parasomnias. Continuum (Minneap Minn) 2017;23:1035–50.

64. Heidbreder A, Frauscher B, Mitterling T, et al. Not only sleepwalking but NREM parasomnia irrespective of the type is associated with HLA DQB1*05:01. J Clin Sleep Med 2016;12:565–70.

65. Nevsimalova S, Prihodova I, Kemlink D, et al. Childhood parasomnia - a disorder of sleep maturation? Eur J Paediatr Neuro 2013;17:615–9.

66. Pressman MR. Factors that predispose, prime and precipitate NREM parasomnias in adults: clinical and forensic implications. Sleep Med Rev 2007;11:5–30.

67. Zadra A, Pilon M, Montplaisir J. Polysomnographic diagnosis of sleepwalking: effects of sleep deprivation. Ann Neurol 2008;63:513–9.

68. Larsen CH, Dooley J, Gordon K. Fever-associated confusional arousal. Eur J Pediatr 2004;163:696–7.

69. Lopez R, Jaussent I, Scholz S, et al. Functional impairment in adult sleepwalkers: a case-control study. Sleep 2013;36:345–51.

70. Molina AT. Parasomnias: common sleep disorders in children suffering from obstructive sleep apnea syndrome. Medisur-Rev Cienc Me 2010;8:437–44.

71. Gurbani N, Dye TJ, Dougherty K, et al. Improvement of parasomnias after treatment of restless leg syndrome/periodic limb movement disorder in children. J Clin Sleep Med 2019;15:743–8.

72. Pressman MR. Sleepwalking, Amnesia, comorbid conditions and triggers: effects of recall and other methodological biases. Sleep 2013;36:1757–8.

73. Mindell JA, Barrett KM. Nightmares and anxiety in elementary-aged children: is there a relationship. Child Care Health Dev 2002;28:317–22.

74. Stein MA, Mendelsohn J, Obermeyer WH, et al. Sleep and behavior problems in school-aged children. Pediatrics 2001;107(4):E60.

75. Schredl M, Biemelt J, Roos K, et al. Nightmares and stress in children. Sleep and hypnosis 2008;10:19–25.

76. Nielsen TA, Laberge L, Paquet J, et al. Development of disturbing dreams during adolescence

and their relation to anxiety symptoms. Sleep 2000; 23:727–36.

77. Schredl M, Reinhard I. Gender differences in nightmare frequency: a meta-analysis. Sleep Med Rev 2011;15:115–21.

78. Hublin C, Kaprio J, Partinen M, et al. Nightmares: familial aggregation and association with psychiatric disorders in a nationwide twin cohort. Am J Med Genet 1999;88:329–36.

79. Solms M. Dreaming and REM sleep are controlled by different brain mechanisms. Behav Brain Sci 2000;23:843–50. discussion 904-1121.

80. Gieselmann A, Ait Aoudia M, Carr M, et al. Aetiology and treatment of nightmare disorder: state of the art and future perspectives. J Sleep Res 2019;28:e12820.

81. Germain A, Buysse DJ, Nofzinger E. Sleep-specific mechanisms underlying posttraumatic stress disorder: integrative review and neurobiological hypotheses. Sleep Med Rev 2008;12:185–95.

82. Nielsen T. The stress Acceleration Hypothesis of nightmares. Front Neurol 2017;8:201.

83. Thompson A, Lereya ST, Lewis G, et al. Childhood sleep disturbance and risk of psychotic experiences at 18: UK birth cohort. Br J Psychiat 2015; 207:23–9.

84. Liu XC, Liu ZZ, Chen RH, et al. Nightmares are associated with future suicide attempt and non-suicidal self-injury in adolescents. J Clin Psychiat 2019;80(4):18m12181.

85. Bloomfield ER, Shatkin JP. Parasomnias and movement disorders in children and adolescents. Child Adol Psych Cl 2009;18:947.

86. Rousseau A, Belleville G. The mechanisms of action underlying the efficacy of psychological nightmare treatments: a systematic review and thematic analysis of discussed hypotheses. Sleep Med Rev 2018;39:122–33.

87. Augedal AW, Hansen KS, Kronhaug CR, et al. Randomized controlled trials of psychological and pharmacological treatments for nightmares: a meta-analysis. Sleep Med Rev 2013;17:143–52.

88. Simard V, Nielsen T. Adaptation of imagery rehearsal therapy for nightmares in children: a brief report. Psychotherapy 2009;46:492–7.

89. Allen RP, Picchietti D, Hening WA, et al. Restless legs syndrome: diagnostic criteria, special considerations, and epidemiology. A report from the restless legs syndrome diagnosis and epidemiology workshop at the National Institutes of Health. Sleep Med 2003;4:101–19.

90. Picchietti DL, Bruni O, de Weerd A, et al. Pediatric restless legs syndrome diagnostic criteria: an update by the International restless legs syndrome study group. Sleep Med 2013;14:1253–9.

91. Picchietti D, Allen RP, Walters AS, et al. Restless legs syndrome: prevalence and impact in children and adolescents - the Peds REST study. Pediatrics 2007;120:253–66.

92. Turkdogan D, Bekiroglu N, Zaimoglu S. A prevalence study of restless legs syndrome in Turkish children and adolescents. Sleep Med 2011;12:315–21.

93. Chervin RD, Archbold KH, Dillon JE, et al. Associations between symptoms of inattention, hyperactivity, restless legs, and periodic leg movements. Sleep 2002;25:213–8.

94. Walters AS, Hickey K, Maltzman J, et al. A questionnaire study of 138 patients with restless legs syndrome: the 'Night-Walkers' survey. Neurology 1996;46:92–5.

95. Zhang JH, Lam SP, Li SX, et al. Restless legs symptoms in adolescents: epidemiology, heritability, and pubertal effects. J Psychosom Res 2014;76: 158–64.

96. Jimenez-Jimenez FJ, Alonso-Navarro H, Garcia-Martin E, et al. Genetics of restless legs syndrome: an update. Sleep Med Rev 2018;39:108–21.

97. Khan FH, Ahlberg CD, Chow CA, et al. Iron, dopamine, genetics, and hormones in the pathophysiology of restless legs syndrome. J Neurol 2017; 264:1634–41.

98. Beard JL. Iron status and periodic limb movements of sleep in children: a causal relationship? Sleep Med 2004;5:89–90.

99. Angriman M, Cortese S, Bruni O. Somatic and neuropsychiatric comorbidities in pediatric restless legs syndrome: a systematic review of the literature. Sleep Med Rev 2017;34:34–45.

100. Simakajornboon N, Dye TJ, Walters AS. Restless legs syndrome/Willis-Ekbom disease and growing pains in children and adolescents. Sleep Med Clin 2015;10:311.

101. DelRosso L, Bruni O. Chapter Eleven - treatment of pediatric restless legs syndrome. In: Clemens S, Ghorayeb I, editors. Advances in Pharmacology, 84. Academic Press; 2019. p. 237–53.

102. Walters AS, Mandelbaum DE, Lewin DS, et al. Dopaminergic therapy in children with restless legs/periodic limb movements in sleep and ADHD. Pediatr Neurol 2000;22:182–6.

103. Allen RP, Picchietti DL, Auerbach M, et al. Evidence-based and consensus clinical practice guidelines for the iron treatment of restless legs syndrome/ Willis-Ekbom disease in adults and children: an IRLSSG task force report. Sleep Med 2018;41:27–44.

104. Mindell JA, Sadeh A, Wiegand B, et al. Co-sleeping, parental presence, and sleep in young children: a cross-cultural perspective. Sleep 2009;32:A81–2.

105. Latz S, Wolf AW, Lozoff B. Cosleeping in context - sleep practices and problems in young children in Japan and the United States. Arch Pediat Adol Med 1999;153:339–46.

106. Liu X, Liu L, Owens JA, et al. Sleep patterns and sleep problems among schoolchildren in the United States and China. Pediatrics 2005;115:241–9.

107. Kamara D, Beauchaine TP. A review of sleep disturbances among infants and children with neurodevelopmental disorders. Rev J Autism Dev Dis 2020;7:278–94.

108. Cortese S, Faraone SV, Konofal E, et al. Sleep in children with attention-deficit/hyperactivity disorder: meta-analysis of subjective and objective studies. J Am Acad Child Psy 2009;48:894–908.

109. Robinson-Shelton A, Malow BA. Sleep disturbances in neurodevelopmental disorders. Curr Psychiat Rep 2016;18(1):6.

110. Keogh S, Bridle C, Siriwardena NA, et al. Effectiveness of non-pharmacological interventions for insomnia in children with Autism Spectrum Disorder: a systematic review and meta-analysis. Plos One 2019;14(8):e0221428.

111. Blackmer AB, Feinstein JA. Management of sleep disorders in children with neurodevelopmental disorders: a review. Pharmacotherapy 2016;36:84–98.

65   Sleep Complaints Among School Children

Insomnia: Focus on Children

Montida Veeravigrom, MD[a], Weerasak Chonchaiya, MD[b],*

KEYWORDS

- Insomnia • Sleep disturbance • Behavioral management • Children • Adolescence
- Neurodevelopmental disorder

KEY POINTS

- Prevalence of insomnia is often underestimated in primary care pediatric practice and the rate of such a problem is likely to be increasing, particularly during the COVID-19 pandemic.
- Cognitive-behavioral therapy (CBT) and other behavioral interventions are the mainstay for the management of pediatric insomnia.
- There is no FDA-approved medication for insomnia treatment in children.

INTRODUCTION

Insomnia is one of the chief complaints that is common in pediatric practice for pediatricians and pediatric sleep medicine. Children's sleep has integral developmental changes in all aspects. Sleep process, one of the aspects, changes through the maturity of the central nervous system and circadian rhythm across the life span. The concept in diagnosis and evaluation of insomnia is different in each stage of life. Insomnia in children has an impact on the child's self which in turn affects parents' and caretakers' sleep. On the other hand, conflict in the family can be the cause of insomnia in a child. When the parent brings the child to the clinic because of insomnia, most of the symptoms have been ongoing for quite some time and the family may have already tried a few methods on their own, by recommendations from friends or the Internet. Insomnia can also be the symptom of sleep disorders such as obstructive sleep apnea, restless leg syndrome, or restless sleep disorder. Children with insomnia need to be evaluated by health care professionals.

In the coronavirus disease 2019 (COVID-19) pandemic years, the pandemic can cause stressful and traumatic events to children, adolescents, and their families. The lockdown during the early COVID-19 pandemic was reported to have an impact on sleep quality and sleep duration of young children aged 3 to 6 years.[1] The lockdown period with online learning increases the stresses on children that have poor attention spans or learning disability. Children are often on the computer screen for long durations with few breaks and have online homework that usually continues after the class session into the evening and nighttime. Among adolescents, online learning screen time may total more than 10 hours per day. When adolescents return to school, sometimes they feel that they have lost their social skills even though they like to interact with people. Intimidating feelings and coping up with peer pressure could precipitate pediatric insomnia in adolescence.

Prevalence

Pediatric insomnia is globally prevalent. Symptoms of insomnia were reported up to 41% based on parental reports in the general pediatric clinic.[2] Its prevalence in countries around the world is varied. The incidence of insomnia also increased in children with neurodevelopmental disabilities such as autism spectrum disorder (ASD), children

Statement of financial support: This work was not supported by any grants and funding sources.

[a] Section of Child Neurology, Department of Pediatrics, The University of Chicago, Biological Sciences, 5841 South Maryland Avenue Room C-526, MC 3055, Chicago, IL, USA; [b] Maximizing Thai Children's Developmental Potential Research Unit, Division of Growth and Development, Department of Pediatrics, King Chulalongkorn Memorial Hospital, Faculty of Medicine, Chulalongkorn University, Sor Kor Building, 11th Floor, 1873 Rama IV. Road, Pathumwan District, Bangkok 10330, Thailand
* Corresponding author.
E-mail address: weerasak.ch@chula.ac.th

Sleep Med Clin 17 (2022) 67–76
https://doi.org/10.1016/j.jsmc.2021.10.004
1556-407X/22/© 2021 Elsevier Inc. All rights reserved.

with chronic headache, or children with attention-deficit/hyperactivity disorder (ADHD).

Factors Affecting Insomnia

There are multiple factors that influence a child's insomnia. The first thing to determine is whether a child waking up at night is abnormal for his/her developmental age. It is normal for a 4-month-old infant to wake up 2 to 3 times at night and the infant is going to start sleeping the whole night at around 6 months of age. During early childhood years, it is very important to teach children how to self-soothe—where such capacity normally begins to develop at 3 months of age. Several factors affecting infantile insomnia are as follows: parenting, feeding, maternal anxiety level, maternal socioeconomic status, etc. The "3P" model of insomnia is shown later in discussion.[3,4]

(1) Predisposing factors: The factors that a child has as the baseline before insomnia develops such as age, sex, genetic predisposition, individuals' developmental status, temperament or personality, psychological styles, or anxiety level, underlying medical or psychiatric conditions.

(2) Precipitating factors: The factors that initially triggered insomnia such as acute events, acute stress, posttraumatic events, parental psychopathology, and poor parent–child interaction.

(3) Perpetuating factors: The factors that maintain insomnia to become habitual such as inadequate sleep hygiene, schoolwork or peer pressure, unrealistic parental expectations on the child's sleep, inappropriate child-rearing practices, negative parenting styles, and lack of consistent discipline. The most common inadequate sleep hygiene practices in children and adolescents are screen time at bedtime, caffeine use, and inappropriate nap time.

DIAGNOSIS

The International Classification of Sleep Disorder-Third Edition (ICSD-3) defined insomnia as a persistent difficulty with sleep initiation, duration, consolidation, or quality that occurs despite adequate opportunity and circumstances for sleep, resulting in some forms of daytime impairment. To establish the diagnosis of insomnia, there need to be 3 components, as listed later in discussion (**Box 1**). Pediatric insomnia can lead to impaired attention, poor academic performance, and behavioral disturbances. Moreover, chronic insomnia was demonstrated to be also associated with impairments in preschoolers' executive function.[5,6]

Box 1
Three components of insomnia
1. Persistent sleep difficulty
2. Adequate sleep opportunity
3. Associated daytime dysfunction

According to the ICSD-3, insomnia is divided into 3 categories as follows:

1. Chronic insomnia disorder: behavioral insomnia of childhood was categorized into this group.
2. Short-term insomnia disorder
3. Other insomnia disorder

Insomnia can be a sleep complaint associated with medical conditions such as gastroesophageal reflux or chronic pain syndrome. If the medical condition is the sole cause of insomnia, the diagnosis of insomnia should not be made separately. Sleep complaints of acute insomnia can be the initial presentation of autoimmune encephalitis or psychiatric disorders. Another common cause of acute insomnia is the use of medications such as decongestants, selective leukotriene receptor antagonists (ie, montelukast), or beta-blockers.

In children and young adults, sleep onset latencies and periods of wakefulness after sleep onset for more than 20 minutes are considered clinically significant sleep disturbances. Even the ICSD-3 abandoned the classification of insomnia in the ICSD-2 such as 6 subtypes of primary insomnia and 5 subtypes of secondary insomnia. However, the approach to determine insomnia categorization, particularly behavioral insomnia of childhood including sleep onset association insomnia or limit-setting insomnia in young children will guide physicians and parents for evaluation and management steps.

Insomnia in adolescence can overlap between delayed sleep-wake phase disorder/type with psychophysiologic insomnia. When an adolescent develops insomnia or nightmares, physicians need to pay attention to find out whether that individual has depression, suicidal thoughts, or physical/psychological abuse.

Pathophysiology subtypes: to use for evaluation and application for behavioral intervention in children and adolescents.

1. *Sleep onset association insomnia*: This type of insomnia usually occurs in infants, toddlers, and preschoolers who cannot self-soothe or learn to sleep by themselves without specific associations or certain conditions. Young

children have difficulty falling asleep or staying asleep or both from inappropriate sleep associations. They are likely to have fears, separation anxiety, or anxiety about sleeping alone. Falling asleep is usually associated with some form of stimulation (eg, rocking, feeding, car ride) or settings (eg, needing parental presence in the bedroom).[3,6]

2. *Limit setting insomnia*: This type of insomnia usually occurs in preschoolers and older children whereby age-appropriate oppositional behaviors such as bedtime resistance are very common in this age group. Children often refuse to go to bed by showing resistance, verbal protests, or demands to do something else before bed to delay their bedtimes. Children's separation anxiety may result in resistance at bedtime and night wakings.[3] This setting usually occurs when parents have inconsistent limits or implement discipline in an unpredictable manner. As such, the child's sleep onset is ultimately delayed from his or her appropriate schedule.

3. *Psychophysiologic insomnia*: This type of insomnia usually occurs in older children and adolescents. Individuals with psychophysiologic insomnia often have mind racing/ruminating thoughts when they try to fall asleep. They often check the time at night when they cannot fall asleep which in turn makes them have negative thoughts about their performance the next day if they are unable to fall asleep. There is heightening of arousal and learned sleep preventing associations. These children usually sleep better during vacations or at a novel place or when they do not try to sleep.[3]

PEDIATRIC INSOMNIA IN SPECIAL CIRCUMSTANCE
Adolescence

Insomnia in adolescents is relatively common as there are normal physiologic changes in their sleep patterns at this age: sleep onset and offset time are generally delayed related to adolescents' pubertal changes, known as puberty-mediated phase delay.[7] Additionally, sleep–wake patterns are relatively irregular in adolescents. Such changes in adolescents' sleep usually co-occur with other precipitating and perpetuating factors, especially environmental influences including academic and extracurricular demands, peer pressure, earlier required wake times (ie, school start time), discrepancies between bedtimes and wake times for school nights and nonschool nights, and also for the days adolescents have traditional studying at school versus online learning at home during the COVID-19 pandemic in addition to the prolonged use of electronic screen media.[1,7–9] A concurrence of these factors could lead to further delay in both bedtime and wake time and ultimately result in insufficient sleep duration or sleep loss.[7–9] Sleep restriction could impair adolescents' learning, memory, cognitive ability, emotional regulation, and put adolescents at risk for risk-taking behaviors including cigarettes smoking, recreational drug use, unprotected sexual intercourse, injuries related to transport and road safety, violence, psychiatric problems, and suicidality.[8–12] Adolescents aged 13 to 18 years often require 8 to 10 hours of sleep according to the recommendation on the amount of sleep for the pediatric population,[13] but most of them actually sleep less. Although adolescents are likely to oversleep on the weekend to compensate for their chronic tiredness and fatigue from inadequate sleep during weekdays, deficits in their performance, attention, cognitive function, and emotional control from chronic sleep insufficiency still exist.[7,8] Such a habit of weekend oversleeping is reflective of poor sleep hygiene which further triggers adolescents to have more sleep phase delay and results in increased insomnia, sleep disturbances, and circadian disruption.[7,8] Delaying school start time to 8:30 AM or later in middle to high schools demonstrated an increase of total sleep time to 25 to 77 minutes during weekdays and reduction in students' daytime sleepiness.[8,14,15] Moreover, improvement in academic and health outcomes including remaining awake in class, improved class attendance and academic performance, together with lower rates of depressed mood, caffeine consumption, and motor vehicle accidents were also reported.[8,14,15]

Electronic screen media use has become ubiquitous in children and adolescents of all ages. Trends of screen media exposure have been rapidly increasing over the decades, particularly with new digital technology, online learning, and the COVID-19 era. Sleep problems are some of the outcomes which have been shown to be associated with excessive and inappropriate screen media exposure.[16–18] Such sleep difficulties in children and adolescents included later bedtime, delayed sleep onset, shorter sleep duration and total sleep time, daytime sleepiness, and poorer sleep quality.[16–21] Risk factors for developing sleep problems in those exposed to electronic screen media including screen media use at bedtime, in the bedroom; portable devices with violent content; using media in the background; media multitasking; and interactive use, for example, video games and mobile devices.[16–21] There are plausible mechanisms for screen media effects on sleep problems including the displacement of sleep time due to later bedtime; alerting, psychological arousal from entertainment and violent programs and video games; circadian effects of blue light exposure from screen media devices and melatonin suppression.[16,19–21]

Children with Neurodevelopmental Disorders

Insomnia and sleep difficulties in children with neurodevelopmental disorders including ADHD, ASD, intellectual disability (ID), and known genetic syndromes for example, Smith–Magenis syndrome, Angelman syndrome, Rett syndrome, Williams syndrome, Down syndrome, and so forth are more prevalent.[3,22–24] The insomnia in these populations seem to be chronic, more severe, and occur more frequently than that of typically developing children.[3] The prevalence of sleep problems in those with ADHD, ASD, and ID is approximately 30% to 86%.[3,24–29] Individuals with ADHD had significantly higher scores on all subscales of the Children's Sleep Habits Questionnaire (CSHQ) reported by parents including bedtime resistance, sleep duration, sleep anxiety, night waking, parasomnias, sleep-disordered breathing, daytime sleepiness, delayed sleep onset, and total difficulties score on the CSHQ than their counterparts.[22] Furthermore, children with ADHD are more likely to have restless leg syndrome and periodic limb movement disorder.[3] Likewise, those with ASD were more likely to have longer sleep onset latency, bedtime resistance, sleep anxiety, night waking, and total difficulties score reported by their parents than typically developing children.[23] Other sleep disturbances in those with ASD included irregular sleep-wake patterns, decreased sleep efficiency, insufficient total sleep duration, early morning waking, increased daytime sleepiness, obstructive sleep apnea, parasomnias, and periodic limb movement disorder.[24,27] Although higher rates of insomnia and sleep problems in those with neurodevelopmental disorders are observed, such problems are often overlooked by health care providers, particularly in busy clinical settings. If left unrecognized and untreated, inadequate sleep duration and poor sleep quality from such problems could exacerbate more core symptoms, behavioral, emotional, academic, and cognitive problems in addition to poor daily functioning in those with neurodevelopmental disorders, which in turn affect not only the quality of life of affected individuals but also their families.[24,27] Behavioral problems due to insomnia and insufficient sleep in those with neurodevelopmental disorders

include increased ADHD symptoms, more restricted and repetitive behaviors, aggressive and self-injurious behaviors, temper tantrums, and other disruptive behaviors.[24] If children with neurodevelopmental disorders have a new onset of, or a significant exacerbation of individuals' status, and unexplained behavioral problems including irritability, aggression, and self-injurious behaviors; medical problems, especially sleep difficulties and insomnia should be detected early and properly treated.[24] As a result, clinicians should be aware of bidirectional relationships between sleep difficulties and symptoms of neurodevelopmental disorders; therefore, insomnia and sleep problems should both be appropriately addressed and managed.

There are several plausible mechanisms related to a biopsychosocial model which attempt to explain why those with neurodevelopmental disorders have an increased risk of insomnia. Such a model could also be demonstrated as the "3P" model mentioned above for those with neurodevelopmental disorders. Predisposing factors include biological and genetic abnormalities related to individuals' underlying neurodevelopmental disorders and genetic syndromes resulting in disruption in sleep architecture,[30] disturbances in circadian rhythms, sleep/wake cycle consolidation,[31] clock gene abnormalities, melatonin production and secretion, and mutations of circadian-relevant genes in addition to several neurotransmitters' dysregulation.[32,33] Predisposing factors of insomnia in such a population also include the core symptoms of specific neurodevelopmental disorders (inattention, hyperactivity, and impulsivity in those with ADHD; persistent impairments in social communication and social interaction in addition to restricted, repetitive patterns of behaviors or interests in those with ASD) and individuals' cognitive and adaptive functioning. Comorbid or associated conditions occurring with neurodevelopmental disorders including comorbid oppositional defiant behaviors in those with ADHD, comorbid ADHD in those with ASD, learning problems, intellectual impairment, sensory integration problems, and mood disorders could put those with neurodevelopmental disorders at greater risks of insomnia and sleep disturbances. Precipitating factors that could trigger insomnia in those with neurodevelopmental disorders may include concurrent medical illnesses co-occurring with neurodevelopmental disorders for example, seizures, gastroesophageal reflux, constipation, medication use, particularly psychostimulants, atypical antipsychotics, antihistamines, and so forth that could affect the child's sleep pattern—quantity and quality, family stresses, changes in child-rearing practices, routines, and excessive electronic screen media exposure, especially during the COVID-19 pandemic.[1,17,18,30,31,34] Perpetuating factors that could maintain insomnia including poor sleep hygiene, inappropriate child-rearing practices such as parental behaviors that help the child to fall asleep at sleep onset or night awakening which are known as sleep-onset associations or problems with limit-setting at bedtime, excessive electronic screen media use, peer influence, schoolwork, and after school activities that are relatively similar to typically developing children. Early identification of such factors in the "3P" model could help clinicians to develop appropriate management plans tailored for each individual.

EVALUATION

Sleep history is a core component for the evaluation of pediatric insomnia. Detailed sleep intake should start from the bedtime schedule and routines on both weekdays and the weekends and last for 24 hours. In addition, bedtime, sleep onset, frequency, and duration of each night waking, snoring, bedwetting, restless sleep, parasomnias, nightmares, nap time, wake time, time when getting out of bed, and total sleep time should be obtained. A sleep diary and sleep log can be used to obtain individuals' sleep-wake patterns and practices within a 2-week period. Specific sleep disturbances including difficulty initiating, staying asleep, and problems sleeping without caregiver's intervention, bedtime resistance, and waking up earlier than desired time should be thoroughly elicited. Associated daytime symptoms such as impairments in social and family interaction, academic performance, daytime sleepiness, inattention, behavioral, and emotional problems, and so forth should also be ascertained. Moreover, inadequate opportunity and circumstances for sleep in addition to other potential sleep disorders (ie, obstructive sleep apnea, delayed sleep-phase disorder, restless leg syndrome, etc.) should be ruled out before making the diagnosis of chronic insomnia disorder. Other histories, especially predisposing factors (ie, underlying medical and psychiatric disorders); precipitating factors (ie, anxiety, acute stresses, and posttraumatic events that individuals have experienced), and perpetuating factors (ie, parenting practices, parental responses to the child at bedtime and night waking, sleep hygiene, schoolwork, peer pressure, screen media exposure, caffeine use, medications, smoking, drug and alcohol use, etc.) should be comprehensively evaluated to guide in making the diagnosis and plan for further management.

Furthermore, sleep questionnaires can be used clinically to screen for sleep problems in pediatric individuals at health supervision visits. BEARS sleep screening tool (**Box 2**) can be used for a wide age range. However, the questions may need to be adjusted according to the patient's sleep physiology.[7,35] Excessive daytime sleepiness during preschool and school age may manifest as sleeping during the car ride or taking naps longer than a normal child at that age. The CSHQ is another sleep questionnaire commonly used to assess sleep behaviors and difficulties in preschool- and school-aged children in both research and clinical settings.[36] Parents or caregivers are required to rate sleep behaviors of their children in a recent typical week based on a 3-point Likert scale; 1) "usually" if sleep behaviors occurred 5–7 times per week, 2) "sometimes" for behaviors that occurred 2–4 times a week, and 3) "rarely" if behaviors occurred only 0 to 1 time per week. The CSHQ comprises 8 subscales including bedtime resistance, sleep duration, sleep anxiety, night waking, parasomnias, sleep-disordered breathing, daytime sleepiness, and sleep-onset delay which are computed to determine a total difficulties score. Higher scores are indicative of sleep difficulties in each subscale as well as the total score. These questionnaires may be included as intake forms for an initial evaluation of sleep difficulties in some settings.

Actigraphy is beneficial in evaluating insomnia when sleep diaries are not reliable. Sleep diaries tend to overestimate the sleep time and underestimate the wake after sleep onset time. Actigraphy will also help in establishing the diagnosis of delayed sleep–wake phase disorder in adolescents who present with the complaint of insomnia. Polysomnography is useful in determining the presence of any other sleep disorder that can cause the complaint of insomnia such as obstructive sleep apnea, periodic limb movement disorder, or if the patient has paradoxical insomnia.

BEHAVIORAL MANAGEMENT OF INSOMNIA

Behavioral intervention is essential and should be the first step for the management of insomnia,

---

Box 2
BEARS sleep screening tool[35]

*B*edtime problems

*E*xcessive daytime sleepiness

*A*wakenings during the night

*R*egularity and duration of sleep

*S*leep-disordered breathing

particularly in the pediatric population. Behavioral management not only improves children's sleep quantity, quality, and regularity, but also minimizes ADHD symptoms, daytime problematic behaviors, and mood problems in addition to improving the quality of life in both typically developing children and those with neurodevelopmental disorders.[12,25,37] Moreover, improvements in parental mood, stress, competence, and well-being were also observed.[3] Behavioral management should start with psychoeducation about the specific diagnosis of pediatric insomnia to help parents and caregivers better understand the nature of children's insomnia symptoms and factors affecting insomnia. For instance, sleep onset association insomnia is caused by infants' inability to self-soothe or self-regulate at sleep onset without specific conditions, whereas limit setting insomnia occurs due to parental difficulties in setting limits and managing preschoolers' delaying bedtime behaviors. Psychophysiologic insomnia or primary insomnia is caused by learned sleep-preventing associations and increased arousal at bedtime, particularly in older children and adolescents. Education on regular sleep schedules, bedtime routines, healthy sleep practices, and sleep hygiene should be provided and targeted for all individuals with insomnia to underscore the importance of optimal sleep on a child's health. Sleep-wake schedules, particularly bedtime and wake time for both school nights and nonschool nights should not differ for more than 1 hour. Consistent limits and discipline among each child's caregivers are very important to implement such targets. Sleep hygiene for children and adolescents is displayed in **Box 3**.

Children with sleep onset association insomnia should be trained to self-soothe without certain conditions. They should be put to bed drowsy but awake and gradually weaned from parental presence. If an infant cries and is unable to get back to sleep without certain interventions (ie, rocking, holding, feeding, car riding, etc.), parents need to be very patient with the infant's crying and wait for a few minutes before going to gently pat the infant's buttock or back for brief reassurance without giving the above-mentioned interventions to the child. For every signal or crying from the infant, such parental waiting time should be successively longer, whereas the time a parent assists the infant to go back to sleep should be progressive briefer.[7] Such a behavioral management program using a more gradual withdrawal technique is more acceptable by most parents. However, caregivers should be aware of the possibility of excessive crying or extinction bursts during the implementation of this behavioral management

Box 3
Sleep hygiene for children and adolescents

- Set and maintain regular bedtime routines
- Promote quiet time approximately 30 to 60 minutes before bed
- Promote regular and similar bedtime and wake time every day (no more than 1-hour difference between school nights and nonschool nights)
- Keep the bedroom comfortable, quiet, and dark
- Keep electronic screen media devices out of the bedroom and avoid screen time at least 1 hour before bed
- Use bed for sleeping only
- Spend time outdoors every day and exercise regularly
- Avoid stimulating play and exercise before bedtime
- Avoid hunger, caffeine use, smoking, and alcohol before bed
- Avoid longer naps in the afternoon and after 3:00 PM or 4 hours before bedtime
- Avoid weekend oversleeping
- Avoid using sleeping medications without physician's recommendation

technique.[7] Transitional objects for self-soothing and reduction of separation anxiety during bedtime could also be offered for older infants.[7] Furthermore, positive reinforcement should be initiated if the child is able to sleep by him/herself at sleep onset or after night awakening.

Regarding limit-setting insomnia, appropriate discipline for setting limits and decreased attention for the child's delaying behaviors at bedtime (ie, bedtime resistance, demanding more play, bedtime stories, and going to the toilet, etc.), should be emphasized. Moreover, appropriate bedtime routines should be established. Bedtime should be temporarily set closer to the actual sleep onset, particularly for those with mismatch between parental expectation and the child's circadian rhythm, then the bedtime is gradually advanced earlier.[7] Positive reinforcement such as star charts for desirable bedtime behaviors and remaining in bed, or praise for the child's compliant behaviors at bedtime could be beneficial. Such discipline techniques should be consistently implemented among adults in the same household. Furthermore, relaxation techniques can be used for older children.[7] With respect to psychophysiologic insomnia, the bed should be restricted for actual sleep only. If individuals cannot fall asleep, they should get out of bed for 15 minutes and engage in calming activities in other areas of the house to avoid pairing association between the bed and difficulty falling asleep or anxiety. This is known as stimulus control. Cognitive-behavioral therapy (CBT) is helpful for this type of insomnia to alleviate maladaptive and ruminative thoughts about sleep and its daytime consequences.[4,7,37] CBT is also effective for minimizing perpetuating factors of insomnia, especially psychological and behavioral factors.[4] Relaxation techniques including progressive muscle relaxation, diaphragmatic breathing, and visual imagery should be included as a behavioral management plan to reduce individuals' anxiety.[4,38] CBT has been shown to improve sleep onset latency, wake after sleep onset, and sleep efficiency more than other symptoms.[37,38]

PHARMACOLOGICAL MANAGEMENT OF INSOMNIA

Behavioral management is the mainstay of insomnia management. Medical treatment should be considered the second line when behavioral management is not effective. Medication treatment should not be the sole management of insomnia in children. The most effective strategy is to combine pharmacologic and behavioral management. Other points are to maintain the sustainability of treatment and decrease side effects. Physicians should start medication after detailed history and physical examination, with the benefits outweighing the risks. Currently, there is no medication approved by the United States Food and Drug Administration (USFDA) for insomnia treatment. Relative contraindications to pharmacologic treatment of children with insomnia are displayed in **Box 4**.

Great consideration should be practiced when starting sedative/hypnotic medication in adolescents. For children, physicians should practice extreme caution if there is underlying depression, especially when using medication with high toxicity, as there is a risk of overdosage.

Box 4
Relative contraindications to pharmacologic treatment of children with insomnia

- Insomnia caused by self-limiting conditions (eg, teething)
- Current alcohol or illicit substance abuse
- Inadequate chance to monitor side-effects or for follow-up

Melatonin

Melatonin is the endogenous hormone from the pineal gland which is secreted during darkness and is suppressed by light. Melatonin has both chronobiotic (to move the body clock) and hypnotic properties. There is evidence for its use in delayed sleep-wake phase disorder and decreased sleep latency in children with sleep-onset insomnia. The mechanism of action is through MT1 and/or MT2 receptors.[39,40] Melatonin is one of the most common drugs that pediatricians use for children and adolescents with sleep disturbances.[41] Melatonin has been used in typically developing children and children with ADHD, ASD, and other neurodevelopmental disabilities. It is also useful in sleep disturbance in children with genetic syndromes such as Smith–Magenis syndrome, Angelman syndrome, Rett syndrome, and tuberous sclerosis.[40,42] For pharmacokinetics, melatonin has low bioavailability with intense hepatic first-pass metabolism particularly the CYP1A2 which may determine high or low metabolizers.[43]

Melatonin has 2 forms in terms of duration of action with immediate-release and extended-release melatonin. Immediate-release or short-acting melatonin is used as a chronobiotic or hypnotic. Melatonin dosage depends on the goal of using it. To use it as a chronobiotic, use a smaller dosage of 0.3 to 0.5 mg. 3 to 5 hours before dim light melatonin onset (DLMO).[39,44] To use for its hypnotic properties, administer 2 hours before bedtime (at that DLMO).[39] The dosages in infants, children, and adolescents are 1 mg., 2 to 3 mg., and 5 mg., respectively.[40,42,45] For extended- or prolonged-release melatonin, European Medicines Agency (EMA) gave positive recommendation under Pediatric Use Marketing Authorization (PUMA) for children and adolescents with ASD and/or Smith–Magenis syndrome in September 2018.[46] The side effects in adolescents are sleep drunkenness or difficulty waking up in the morning.[43]

A recent randomized controlled trial using prolonged-release melatonin nightly for up to 104 weeks for insomnia in children with ASD demonstrated that it was safe and effective. There were no observed side effects on growth and puberty or withdrawal symptoms.[47] The American Academy of Neurology's recent guidelines for insomnia in children with ASD stated that clinicians should offer melatonin if behavioral strategies have not been helpful, and contributing coexisting conditions, or uses of concomitant medication have been addressed. Clinicians should recommend using pharmaceutical grade if available and patients and parents should be counseled about potential side effects of melatonin usage.[27,39]

Melatonin Receptor Agonist

Ramelteon is the potent selective dual MT1 and MT2 receptor agonist that is the only FDA-approved melatonin preparation for insomnia in adults. There is a case report of ramelteon use in 2 children with ASD.[48] In adults, Ramelteon seemed to work better for insomnia from circadian rhythm abnormality.

Alpha Agonist

Clonidine or guanfacine is an alpha-adrenergic agonist that inhibits norepinephrine release and transmission by acting on presynaptic neurons. It was approved by the FDA for the treatment of hypertension and ADHD.[25] It is also an effective treatment of tics or Tourette syndrome. Clonidine is commonly used by pediatricians and sleep pediatricians for sleep disturbance. Clonidine or guanfacine may be prescribed for insomnia in children with ADHD or Tourette syndrome. The potential adverse side effect is dizziness and hypotension.

Antidepressants

Sedative antidepressants have also been used for insomnia treatment. Histamine (H1) antagonists such as amitriptyline, doxepin, mirtazapine (potent), or trazodone (weak) have a sedative effect. There is a lack of methodology research papers supporting the use of antidepressants for insomnia in children. Sedative antidepressants should be reserved for children with concurrent mood disorder, or chronic migraine headache who use amitriptyline as prophylaxis. Adverse side effects include anticholinergic effects such as dry mouth and urinary retention. For tricyclic antidepressants, there are concerns regarding intoxication and cardiac arrhythmia.

Antihistamine

First-generation antihistamines such as diphenhydramine, cyproheptadine, and hydroxyzine are commonly used medications by pediatricians for sleep disturbance. Pediatricians have confidence in using it for itching or allergy symptoms for extended periods. The first paper regarding the efficacy of diphenhydramine for sleep disorders was 45 years ago.[49] Few research papers on antihistamine for insomnia have been published. An RCT of diphenhydramine in infants did not show greater efficacy compared with placebo in nighttime awakening or overall parental satisfaction.[50] In adults, the American Academy of Sleep Medicine guidelines do not recommend using antihistamine for insomnia. Antihistamine anticholinergic side

effects commonly include dry mouth, urinary retention, blurred vision, constipation, and confusion.

Benzodiazepine and Nonbenzodiazepine Gabaminergic Receptor Agonists

There are 2 randomized controlled trials in children with this type of medication. First, the 8-week multicenter RCT double-blinded placebo trial of Zolpidem failed to reduce sleep latency in children aged 6 to 17 years with ADHD.[51] The most common side effects were headache, dizziness, and hallucination such that 7.4% of the patients discontinued treatment due to adverse effects.[51] Second, an RCT double-blinded placebo trial of eszopiclone was conducted for 12 weeks for insomnia in children aged 6 to 17 years with ADHD.[52] Eszopiclone up to 3 mg. failed to reduce sleep latency.[52] The most frequent emergent side effects were headache, dysgeusia, and dizziness.[52] As such, benzodiazepine and nonbenzodiazepine gabaminergic receptor agonists groups are not good medications for chronic insomnia in children.

Iron Supplement

Ferrous sulfate is the main treatment of restless leg syndrome in children. Ferrous sulfate is also the first-line treatment of the newly categorized entity, restless sleep disorder. In ASD or children with neurodevelopmental disabilities, the parents complain of restless sleep without sensory symptoms of the patient's legs. A recent RCT of ferrous sulfate for insomnia in children with ASD did not show improvement in sleep onset latency and wake after sleep onset time. However, only 20 patients were successfully enrolled.[53]

CLINICS CARE POINTS

- Thorough sleep history is a core component for the evaluation of pediatric insomnia.

- A sleep diary can be used to obtain individuals' sleep-wake patterns and practices within a 2-week period.

- Predisposing, precipitating, and perpetuating factors of insomnia should be comprehensively evaluated to guide in making the diagnosis and plan for further management.

- Education on behavioral management, healthy sleep practices, and sleep hygiene should be provided and targeted toward all pediatric individuals with insomnia.

- Clinicians should offer melatonin if behavioral strategies have not been helpful, and when contributing coexisting conditions, or use of concomitant medication have been addressed.

- To use melatonin as a chronobiotic, a smaller dose of 0.3 to 0.5 mg. is given 3 to 5 hours before dim light melatonin onset (DLMO). To use for its hypnotic properties, administer 1 mg., 2 to 3 mg., and 5 mg. 2 hours before bedtime (at that DLMO) for infants, children, and adolescents, respectively.

DISCLOSURE

The authors have nothing to disclose.

REFERENCES

1. Dellagiulia A, Lionetti F, Fasolo M, et al. Early impact of COVID-19 lockdown on children's sleep: a 4-week longitudinal study. J Clin Sleep Med 2020;16(9): 1639–40.

2. Archbold KH, Pituch KJ, Panahi P, et al. Symptoms of sleep disturbances among children at two general pediatric clinics. J Pediatr 2002;140(1):97–102.

3. Owens JA, Mindell JA. Pediatric insomnia. Pediatr Clin North Am 2011;58(3):555–69.

4. Himelfarb M, Shatkin JP. Pediatric insomnia. Child Adolesc Psychiatr Clin N Am 2021;30(1):117–29.

5. Bruni O, Melegari MG, Esposito A, et al. Executive functions in preschool children with chronic insomnia. J Clin Sleep Med 2020;16(2):231–41.

6. American Academy of Sleep Medicine. ICSD-3). In: The International classification of sleep disorders –. Third edition. Westchester: American Academy of Sleep Medicine; 2014.

7. Owens JA. Sleep medicine. In: Kliegman RM, Geme JW St, Blum NJ, et al, editors. Nelson textbook of pediatrics. 21st edition. Philadelphia: Elsevier; 2020. p. 172–84.

8. Crowley SJ, Wolfson AR, Tarokh L, et al. An update on adolescent sleep: new evidence informing the perfect storm model. J Adolesc 2018;67:55–65.

9. Tarokh L, Saletin JM, Carskadon MA. Sleep in adolescence: physiology, cognition and mental health. Neurosci Biobehav Rev 2016;70:182–8.

10. Short MA, Weber N. Sleep duration and risk-taking in adolescents: a systematic review and meta-analysis. Sleep Med Rev 2018;41:185–96.

11. Chan NY, Zhang J, Tsang CC, et al. The associations of insomnia symptoms and chronotype with daytime sleepiness, mood symptoms and suicide risk in adolescents. Sleep Med 2020;74:124–31.

12. de Zambotti M, Goldstone A, Colrain IM, et al. Insomnia disorder in adolescence: diagnosis, impact, and treatment. Sleep Med Rev 2018;39: 12–24.

13. Paruthi S, Brooks LJ, D'Ambrosio C, et al. Recommended amount of sleep for pediatric populations: a consensus statement of the American Academy of Sleep Medicine. J Clin Sleep Med 2016;12(6): 785–6.

14. Minges KE, Redeker NS. Delayed school start times and adolescent sleep: a systematic review of the experimental evidence. Sleep Med Rev 2016;28: 86–95.

15. Wheaton AG, Chapman DP, Croft JB. School start times, sleep, behavioral, health, and academic outcomes: a review of the literature. J Sch Health 2016;86(5):363–81.

16. Hale L, Kirschen GW, LeBourgeois MK, et al. Youth screen media habits and sleep: sleep-friendly screen behavior recommendations for clinicians, educators, and parents. Child Adolesc Psychiatr Clin N Am 2018;27(2):229–45.

17. Vijakkhana N, Wilaisakditipakorn T, Ruedeekhajorn K, et al. Evening media exposure reduces night-time sleep. Acta Paediatr 2015;104(3):306–12.

18. Chonchaiya W, Wilaisakditipakorn T, Vijakkhana N, et al. Background media exposure prolongs nighttime sleep latency in Thai infants. Pediatr Res 2017;81(2):322–8.

19. Luyster FS, Strollo PJ Jr, Zee PC, et al. Sleep: a health imperative. Sleep 2012;35(6):727–34.

20. Hysing M, Pallesen S, Stormark KM, et al. Sleep and use of electronic devices in adolescence: results from a large population-based study. BMJ Open 2015;5(1):e006748.

21. Rosen L, Carrier LM, Miller A, et al. Sleeping with technology: cognitive, affective, and technology usage predictors of sleep problems among college students. Sleep Health 2016;2(1):49–56.

22. Chiraphadhanakul K, Jaimchariyatam N, Pruksananonda C, et al. Increased sleep disturbances in Thai children with attention-deficit hyperactivity disorder compared with typically developing children. Behav Sleep Med 2016;14(6):677–86.

23. Inthikoot N, Chonchaiya W. Sleep problems in children with autism spectrum disorder and typical development. Pediatr Int 2021;63(6):649–57.

24. Myers SM, Challman TD. Autism spectrum disorder. In: Voigt RG, Macias MM, Myers SM, et al, editors. Developmental and behavioral pediatrics. 2nd edition. Itasca: American Academy of Pediatrics; 2018. p. 407–75.

25. Bruni O, Angriman M, Calisti F, et al. Practitioner review: treatment of chronic insomnia in children and adolescents with neurodevelopmental disabilities. J Child Psychol Psychiatry 2018;59(5):489–508.

26. Robinson-Shelton A, Malow BA. Sleep disturbances in neurodevelopmental disorders. Curr Psychiatry Rep 2016;18(1):6.

27. Williams Buckley A, Hirtz D, Oskoui M, et al. Practice guideline: treatment for insomnia and disrupted sleep behavior in children and adolescents with autism spectrum disorder: report of the Guideline Development, Dissemination, and Implementation Subcommittee of the American Academy of Neurology. Neurology 2020;94(9):392–404.

28. Ballester P, Richdale AL, Baker EK, et al. Sleep in autism: a biomolecular approach to aetiology and treatment. Sleep Med Rev 2020;54:101357.

29. Meltzer LJ, Wainer A, Engstrom E, et al. Seeing the whole elephant: a scoping review of behavioral treatments for pediatric insomnia. Sleep Med Rev 2021;56:101410.

30. Mazzone L, Postorino V, Siracusano M, et al. The Relationship between sleep problems, neurobiological alterations, core symptoms of autism spectrum disorder, and psychiatric comorbidities. J Clin Med 2018;7(5):102.

31. Geoffray MM, Nicolas A, Speranza M, et al. Are circadian rhythms new pathways to understand autism spectrum disorder? J Physiol Paris 2016; 110(4 Pt B):434–8.

32. Yang Z, Matsumoto A, Nakayama K, et al. Circadian-relevant genes are highly polymorphic in autism spectrum disorder patients. Brain Dev 2016;38(1):91–9.

33. Brown KM, Malow BA. Pediatric insomnia. Chest 2016;149(5):1332–9.

34. Richdale AL, Schreck KA. Sleep problems in autism spectrum disorders: prevalence, nature, & possible biopsychosocial aetiologies. Sleep Med Rev 2009; 13(6):403–11.

35. Owens JA, Dalzell V. Use of the 'BEARS' sleep screening tool in a pediatric residents' continuity clinic: a pilot study. Sleep Med 2005;6(1):63–9.

36. Owens JA, Spirito A, McGuinn M. The Children's Sleep Habits Questionnaire (CSHQ): psychometric properties of a survey instrument for school-aged children. Sleep 2000;23(8):1043–51.

37. Lunsford-Avery JR, Bidopia T, Jackson L, et al. Behavioral treatment of insomnia and sleep disturbances in school-aged children and adolescents. Child Adolesc Psychiatr Clin N Am 2021;30(1):101–16.

38. Badin E, Haddad C, Shatkin JP. Insomnia: the sleeping giant of pediatric public health. Curr Psychiatry Rep 2016;18(5):47.

39. Ekambaram V, Owens J. Medications used for pediatric insomnia. Child Adolesc Psychiatr Clin N Am 2021;30(1):85–99.

40. Bruni O, Alonso-Alconada D, Besag F, et al. Current role of melatonin in pediatric neurology: clinical recommendations. Eur J Paediatr Neurol 2015; 19(2):122–33.

41. Heussler H, Chan P, Price AM, et al. Pharmacological and non-pharmacological management of sleep disturbance in children: an Australian Paediatric Research Network survey. Sleep Med 2013;14(2): 189–94.

42. Cummings C. Melatonin for the management of sleep disorders in children and adolescents. Paediatr Child Health 2012;17(6):331–6.

43. Lalanne S, Fougerou-Leurent C, Anderson GM, et al. Melatonin: from pharmacokinetics to clinical use in autism spectrum disorder. Int J Mol Sci 2021;22(3): 1490.

44. Felt BT, Chervin RD. Medications for sleep disturbances in children. Neurol Clin Pract 2014;4(1):82–7.

45. Andersen IM, Kaczmarska J, McGrew SG, et al. Melatonin for insomnia in children with autism spectrum disorders. J Child Neurol 2008;23(5):482–5.

46. European Medicines Agency Decision. Summary of product characteristics: Slenyto prolonged-release tablets. 2018. Available at: https://www.ema. europa.eu/en/documents/product-information/ slenyto-epar-product-information_en.pdf. Accessed June 06, 2021.

47. Malow BA, Findling RL, Schroder CM, et al. Sleep, growth, and puberty after 2 years of prolonged-release melatonin in children with autism spectrum disorder. J Am Acad Child Adolesc Psychiatry 2021;60(2):252–61.e3.

48. Stigler KA, Posey DJ, McDougle CJ. Ramelteon for insomnia in two youths with autistic disorder. J Child Adolesc Psychopharmacol 2006;16(5):631–6.

49. Russo RM, Gururaj VJ, Allen JE. The effectiveness of diphenhydramine HCl in pediatric sleep disorders. J Clin Pharmacol 1976;16(5–6):284–8.

50. Merenstein D, Diener-West M, Halbower AC, et al. The trial of infant response to diphenhydramine: the TIRED study–a randomized, controlled, patient-oriented trial. Arch Pediatr Adolesc Med 2006; 160(7):707–12.

51. Blumer JL, Findling RL, Shih WJ, et al. Controlled clinical trial of zolpidem for the treatment of insomnia associated with attention-deficit/hyperactivity disorder in children 6 to 17 years of age. Pediatrics 2009;123(5):e770–6.

52. Sangal RB, Blumer JL, Lankford DA, et al. Eszopiclone for insomnia associated with attention-deficit/hyperactivity disorder. Pediatrics 2014;134(4): e1095–103.

53. Reynolds AM, Connolly HV, Katz T, et al. Randomized, placebo-controlled trial of ferrous sulfate to treat insomnia in children with autism spectrum disorders. Pediatr Neurol 2020;104:30–9.

Sleep Disturbances Linked to Genetic Disorders

Rimawati Tedjasukmana, MD, PhD, RPSGT[a,b,*]

KEYWORDS

- Sleep • Sleep disturbance • Sleep regulation • Genetics • Circadian clock

KEY POINTS

- Sleep is a very complex behavior, regulated by processes that have underlying genetical factors.
- However, up till now, no sleep genes are identified.
- Some sleep disturbances are inherited and have underlying genetic factors.
- Sleep disturbances are caused by the interplay of genetic, neurobiological, and environmental factors.

INTRODUCTION

The understanding of sleep remains elusive, it must have an important purpose, as it survived many evolutionary cycles. Genetic factors are surmised to regulate sleep as evidenced by the heritability of sleep traits, specific genetic polymorphisms of these traits, and existence of familial sleep disorders.[1]

Recent studies in human and animal models have uncovered some genetic factors underlying sleep disturbances. However, there are more questions than answers. Studying the genetic factors underlying sleep disturbance will aid in understanding the underlying mechanism of sleep. Identification of the first familial circadian phenotype (familial advanced sleep phase syndrome [FASPS]) in the late 1990s made it possible to begin genetic mapping and cloning of genes or mutations that have strong effects on human circadian timing, thus starting the quest for understanding the genetics of sleep.[2] In this review, an overview of genetical regulation of sleep and genetic factors underlying several sleep disturbances will be presented.

Genetic Factors of Sleep

Although mechanisms regulating sleep are conserved across species from flies to mammals,

studies find that genes regulating sleep remain ambiguous. The probable cause may be that sleep is not one phenotype; there are variabilities in rapid eye movement (REM) and non-REM (NREM) sleep for instance. Diessler and colleagues found more than 300 sleep phenotypes in mice.[3] Sleep is a very complex behavior that is regulated by the circadian rhythm (process C) and homeostatic drive (process S). Process S keeps track of prior sleep-wake history and controls the homeostatic need for sleep, whereas process C sets the time-of-day that sleep preferably occurs.[4]

Circadian rhythm plays a role in sleep regulation, especially in sleep timing. In mammals, the circadian clock genes consist of activators CLOCK and BMAL1, repressors PER (period) and CRY (cryptochrome).[5] The mechanism consists of clock proteins that regulate their own transcription in an autoregulatory feedback loop.[1,6] The degradation of PER and CRY proteins is also regulated by the serine/threonine kinases, casein kinase 1δ (CK1δ) and CK1ε, the F-box proteins, FBXL3 and FBXL21. Several additional genes and feedback loops have been uncovered, increasing the complexity of the mammalian circadian clock gene network. In a second feedback loop, CLOCK and BMAL1 also regulate the transcription of genes for the nuclear receptors REV-ERBα and REV-ERBβ. A third feedback loop is mediated by

a Department of Neurology, Universitas Kristen Krida Wacana (Krida Wacana Christian University), Jakarta, Indonesia; b Medistra Hospital, Jl. Gatot Subroto Kav 59, Jakarta 12950, Indonesia
* Medistra Hospital, Jl. Gatot Subroto Kav 59, Jakarta 12950, Indonesia
E-mail address: rima.tedja@gmail.com

Sleep Med Clin 17 (2022) 77–86
https://doi.org/10.1016/j.jsmc.2021.10.005
1556-407X/22/© 2021 Elsevier Inc. All rights reserved.

CLOCK/BMAL1-mediated transcription of the gene DBP and the ROR/REV-ERB-mediated transcription of *Nfil3*[7] (**Fig. 1**).

Sleep homeostasis is a process where sleep need accumulates during wakefulness and decreases during sleep. Both circadian rhythm and sleep homeostasis regulate sleep. However, the differences between these 2 processes are not clear cut. The clock genes NPAS2 and CLOCK are sleep-wake driven and not circadian. It was discovered also that sleep deprivation can cause long-term dampening of clock genes expression.[8,9] A variation of PER3 gene is associated with sleep deprivation.[10] Franken and colleagues discovered that PER1, PER2, and DBP are implicated in sleep homeostasis.[4,11] Clock genes also act as sensors of homeostasis in peripheral tissues.[4] These findings suggest that circadian rhythm and sleep homeostasis are closely interlocked. Sleep homeostasis is also caused by build-up and decay of adenosine, which is regulated by 2 genes, the Adora1 and Adk. These genes, respectively, encode the adenosine receptor and its metabolizing enzyme.[12] In conclusion, both processes S and C are genetically regulated.

To make matters even more complicated, other genes also regulate sleep. Voltage-gated potassium channels have a major function in sleep. A genetic screen in *Drosophila* by Cirelli and colleagues identified sleep-inhibiting effects of mutations in the Shaker potassium channel.[13] Also, injury or infection may increase sleep, and some immune genes are involved in sleep promotion. The cytokines IL-1 and TNFα play a role in sleep physiology.[1,14,15] Nuclear factor-κB (NF-κB) increases after sleep deprivation,[16] and Williams and colleagues discovered in *Drosophila* that the immune gene Relish (encoding the Drosophila NF-κB) plays a role in the control of sleep.[17] The EEG features of sleep can also be modulated by the genes that regulate the duration and timing of sleep. DEC2 Y362H mutation carriers showed higher delta power during NREM and less REM sleep compared with the noncarriers.[2] Slow-wave activity in NREM sleep, theta and alpha activity during wakefulness, and REM sleep were all increased in PER3$^{5/5}$ compared with PER3$^{4/4}$ individuals.[10]

Sleep appears to be genetically regulated. However, it is clear from all these observations that despite the increasing number of studies we still cannot elucidate "sleep genes."

Genetic Factors Underlying Narcolepsy and Other Hypersomnia Disorders

Narcolepsy is a chronic neurologic sleep disorder that manifests as a difficulty in maintaining

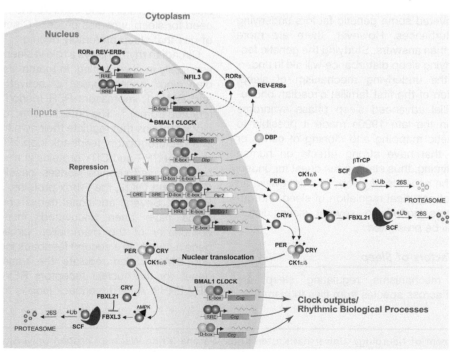

Fig. 1. Components of the mammalian circadian clock. The mammalian clock consisted of 3 feedback loops of clock genes (see text). (*From* Cox KH, Takahashi JS. Circadian clock genes and the transcriptional architecture of the clock mechanism. Journal of Molecular Endocrinology. 2019;63(4):R93-R102. https://doi.org/10.1530/JME-19-0153; with permission.)

continuous wakefulness and sleep. Narcolepsy type 1 (NT1) is characterized by excessive daytime sleepiness, cataplexy, hypnagogic/hypnopompic hallucinations, and sleep paralysis. It is caused by a marked reduction in neurons in the hypothalamus that produce orexin (hypocretin), which is a wakefulness-associated neuropeptide. Narcolepsy type 2 (NT2) has the same symptoms as NT1 excluding cataplexy and has normal cerebrospinal fluid (CSF) hypocretin.[18]

In animal models, this disease can be reproduced by disrupting hypocretin (orexin) transmission by defects in either the hypocretin receptor 2 (HCRTR2) or the hypocretin ligand genes.[19,20] However, it is a different story in human narcolepsy. Although the link between hypocretin deficiency and narcolepsy is consistent in both humans and animal models, the mechanisms underlying the dysfunction are different.[21] Human narcolepsy is sporadic, there is low concordance in monozygotic twins (25%–30%), and only 1% to 2% of first-degree relatives of an NT1 patient have the same disease. However, the relative risk for first-degree family members of patients with NT1 is 10- to 40-fold higher than that in the general population.[22] Narcolepsy is a very complex disease with both genetical and environmental factors. Recent studies have identified susceptibility loci for NT1, but genetical analysis of NT2 is still progressing.[21]

There is hypocretin deficiency in the CSF of NT1 patients. Hypocretin 1 (orexin A) and hypocretin 2 (orexin B) are neuropeptides that control wakefulness and appetite. They are produced by neurons in the lateral hypothalamus.[23,24] However, unlike canine narcolepsy models, most human NT1 patients do not have variants in the prepro-orexin and orexin receptor genes.[21] Loss of hypocretin neurons is probably caused by autoimmune pathology. This fact is apparent by the close association between human leukocyte antigen (HLA) and T cell receptor (TCR) variants of narcolepsy. HLA class II antigens in immune cells present foreign peptides to T cells via TCR. Nearly all NT1 cases carry HLA-DQB1*06:02 gene allele[25] and also 30% to 50% of NT2 cases.[26] The problem is that this is a very common allele in general population and thus is not sufficient as a cause of disease.[27]

Recent data from H1N1 influenza infection and vaccination suggests narcolepsy can develop by interaction between HLA and an immune trigger. Increased prevalence of NT1 was discovered after H1N1 infection in Chinese children[28] and after anti-H1N1 vaccination in European countries.[29,30] On the other hand, genome-wide association (GWA) studies found single-nucleotide polymorphism (SNP) rs5770917 located between CPT1B (carnitine palmitoyltransferase 1B) and CHKB (Choline Kinase B) was associated with NT1. CPT1B regulates β-oxidation, a pathway involved in regulating theta frequency during REM sleep, and CHKB is an enzyme involved in the metabolism of choline, a precursor of the REM- and wake-regulating neurotransmitter acetylcholine.[31] So, either of these genes is a plausible candidate for the development of narcolepsy.

Idiopathic hypersomnia is clinically difficult to differentiate with NT2. The frequency of DQB1*0602 (40%) in patients with idiopathic hypersomnia is intermediate between that in the general population (12%–38%) and that in narcolepsy-cataplexy (70%–100%). Idiopathic hypersomnia may be closely linked to narcolepsy, because a narcolepsy polymorphism located between CPT1B and CHKB may be associated with both narcolepsy and hypersomnia in Japanese cohorts.[32]

Kleine-Levin syndrome is a rare disorder characterized by episodes of hypersomnia and cognitive and behavioral changes. This disorder usually affects adolescent males (frequently reported in Ashkenazi Jews), with some family members are also affected. This data suggests that there is a major susceptibility gene and exposure to an unknown environmental trigger.[1]

Genetics of Circadian Rhythm Sleep-Wake Disorders

Circadian rhythm sleep-wake disorder (CRSWD) is defined as a condition that is "caused by alterations of the circadian time keeping system, its entrainment mechanisms, or a misalignment of the endogenous circadian rhythm and the external environment."[33] One disorder has a well-established cause in clock gene mutations, it is the FASPS.

Advanced sleep phase (ASP) is characterized by a phase-advanced circadian sleep-wake rhythm relative to local solar time. It is suspected to be FASPS when ASP is demonstrated in multiple family members. Advanced sleep-wake phase disorder (ASWPD) is defined as a phase advance of the sleep-wake cycle accompanied by a sleep-related complaint. FASPS is a subtype of ASP and overlaps with ASWPD. Prevalence of ASP is 0.33%, FASPS 0.21%, and ASWPD at least 0.04%. Most cases of young-onset ASP were familial.[34]

FASPS patients tend to sleep and wake very early, their melatonin and core body temperature rhythms are advanced by 4 to 6 hours, and their circadian rhythms are 1 hour shorter compared with conventional sleepers. They have defects in phosphorylation of PER2, with mutations identified in both PER2 and Casein Kinase 1 genes (CK1δ).[1,35,36] The FASPS hPER2 S662 G mutation resulted in PER2 being hypophosphorylated by CKI in vitro. Xu and colleagues showed that phosphorylation at S662 leads to increased PER2 transcription and suggest that phosphorylation at another site leads to PER2 degradation.[37]

Contrary to ASWPD patients, individuals with delayed sleep-wake phase disorder (DSWPD) have later sleep and wake onset compared with the rest of the population. They are often sleep deprived because sleep onset is delayed by the biological clock, whereas morning waking time is enforced by the alarm clock and social/work responsibilities.[38] It is common in adolescents and young adults with an estimated prevalence of 7% to 16%. Archer and colleagues reported a length polymorphism in PER3 and PER3 promoter linked to DSWPD.[39,40] However, another study by Osland and colleagues was not able to reproduce these findings.[41] Another study discovered that this disorder was caused by mutation in the core circadian clock gene CRY1 that causes its translation product to constitutively repress the circadian transcriptional activators CLOCK and BMAL1.[42]

Genetics of Restless Legs Syndrome

Restless legs syndrome (RLS)/Willis-Ekbom disease is characterized by an urgency to move the legs occurring with abnormal leg sensations. These disturbing sensations can be relieved by movement. These symptoms have a definite circadian presentation; they are worse at night time. The pathophysiology involves iron-dopamine connectivity, iron regulation in the brain, opioid signaling, as well as brain and spinal cord circuitry.[43,44]

Sixty percent of RLS patients reported other family members with this disorder, also there was high concordance (83%) in monozygotic twins.[1,43] GWA studies discovered transcription factors MEIS1, important for nervous system development and affecting dopamine signaling, and BTBD9, which regulates the activity of the striatum.[45,46] MEIS1 is the most important gene involved in RLS pathology. This gene is expressed in dopaminergic neurons of the substantia nigra, the spinal cord, and the red nucleus (regulates coordination of limb movement and that also contains lower iron levels in RLS). MEIS1 is part of a regulatory network that specifies motor neuron pool identity and the pattern of target-muscle connectivity.[1] BTBD9 regulates striatal activity. Recent studies suggest that changes in the striatum may underlie the pathogenesis of RLS.[47] Brain imaging studies show decreased striatal dopamine transporter[48] and D_2 dopamine receptor binding potential.[49] Also, this gene is associated with periodic limb movement in sleep, inferring that it is important for the motor symptoms of RLS.[50]

GWA studies also discovered a third locus containing the genes encoding mitogen-activated protein kinase MAP2K5 and the transcription factor SKOR1(LBXCOR1) on chromosomes 2p, 6p, and 15q, respectively.[45] SKOR1 is expressed selectively in a subset of dorsal horn interneurons in the developing spinal cord, which relay pain and touch. This locus may contribute to the sensory component of RLS by affecting modulation of sensory and pain inputs.

Genetics of Insomnia

Insomnia is characterized with persistent difficulty in initiating or maintaining sleep, with corresponding daytime dysfunction. It occurs in 10% to 20% of the general population. Insomnia increases the risk of developing anxiety disorders, alcohol abuse, major depression, and cardiometabolic disease.[51] Insomnia runs in families and has higher concordance in monozygotic twins.[1]

GWA studies identified 57 loci for self-reported insomnia symptoms in the UK Biobank, some of them are MEIS1, CYCL1, TMEM132E, and SCFD2. There was evidence of shared genetic factors between frequent insomnia symptoms and RLS, aging, cardiometabolic, behavioral, psychiatric, and reproductive traits. This study also found a possible causal link between insomnia symptoms and coronary artery disease, depressive symptoms and subjective well-being.[51]

Fatal familial insomnia (FFI) is a rare disorder characterized by severe sleep disorder, dysautonomia, motor signs, and abnormal behavior. Primary atrophy of selected thalamic nuclei and inferior olives is usually found in this disorder, and expansion to other brain regions with disease progression. It is an autosomal dominant inherited prion disease caused by D178N mutation in the prion protein gene (PRNP D178N) accompanied by the presence of a methionine at the codon 129 polymorphic site on the mutated allele.[52,53] Loss of sleep, sympathetic hyperactivity, and flattening of vegetative and hormonal circadian oscillations characterize FFI. These symptoms resulted from homeostatic imbalance caused by the interruption of the thalamocortical limbic circuits, the phylogenetically most advanced structures involved in the control of the sleep-wake cycle and the body's homeostasis.[54]

Short sleeper is usually classified under the heading of insomnia as isolated symptoms and normal variants.[33] Familial natural short sleeper is an extreme early bird phenotype. Similar to individuals with FASPS, they wake up at an extremely early hour in the morning. However, their sleep onset time was comparable to conventional sleepers, thus shortening their total sleep duration by 2 hours each day compared to conventional sleepers. Their sleep time requirement is approximately 6 hours.[38,55] These individuals have a mutation in DEC2, which plays a role in circadian rhythm (as a repressor of CLOCK/BMAL activity[55]) and act as a transcriptional repressor of hypocretin (Hcrt) encoding the neuropeptides HCRT1 and 2[55–57].

Genetics of Sleep-Related Breathing Disorders

Sleep-related breathing disorders (SRBDs) are characterized by abnormalities of respiration during sleep. They may experience repetitive episodes of decreased or arrested respiratory airflow during sleep.[33,58] SRBDs include obstructive sleep apnea (OSA) disorders, central sleep apnea disorders, sleep-related hypoventilation disorders, and sleep-related hypoxemia disorders.[33]

OSA is a syndrome characterized by repetitive upper airway obstruction caused by reduced patency of the upper airway during sleep. OSA is heritable, because first-degree relatives of an OSA patient are more likely to snore or have observed apneas, after controlling for obesity, age, and gender.[59] There is evidence of both direct genetic contributions to OSA susceptibility and indirect contributions via "intermediate" phenotypes such as obesity, craniofacial structure, neurologic control of upper airway muscles and of sleep and circadian rhythm.[60] Approximately 40% of the variance in the apnea-hypopnea index may be explained by familial factors.[61] Studies in twin and family suggest that ventilatory responsiveness to either hypoxemia or hypercapnia, obesity, upper airway dimension, and craniofacial morphology are also under a high degree of genetic control.[62–65]

Despite the evidence of heritability, no risk locus for OSA has reached a genome-wide level of significance. Some studies identified candidate genes for OSA, they are associated with inflammation, hypoxia signaling, and sleep pathways.[58] Polymorphism in the angiopoietin-2 gene (ANGPT2),[66] TNF-α gene,[67] prostaglandin E2 receptor (PTGER3) gene, and lysophosphatidic acid receptor 1 (LPAR1) gene, G-protein receptor gene (GPR83), β-arrestin 1 (ARRB1) gene, an important regulator of hypoxia-inducible factor 1 alpha (HIF-1α), were associated with OSA.[60] In conclusion, OSA is a complex disease, it is probably caused by a combination of many genetic and environmental factors.

Congenital central hypoventilation syndrome (CCHS) or Ondine's curse is a life-threatening disorder involving an impaired ventilatory response to hypercarbia and hypoxemia. It is characterized by alveolar hypoventilation and autonomic dysregulation. Mutations in the paired-like homeobox 2B (PHOX2B) gene underly CCHS. PHOX2B is a master gene for the formation and/or function of the neuronal network for autonomous control of ventilation.[68,69]

Genetics of Sleep Disturbance in Psychiatric Disorders

SNPs in core circadian clock genes have been associated with psychiatric disorders. Several studies have highlighted that circadian clock genes may have a more widespread physiologic effect on cognition, mood, and reward-related behaviors.[70] An SNP in the 3-flanking region of the Clock gene (3111 T to C) is associated with a higher recurrence rate of bipolar episodes. This SNP was also associated in bipolar disorder with sleep problems (insomnia and decreased need for sleep).[71] Several SNPs in the Clock gene (3117 G to T, 3125 A to G) have been reported to be associated with major depression and sleep disturbances.[70] Schizophrenia patients presented disruptions in diurnal rhythms of the expression of PER1, PER2, PER3, and NPAS2 in white blood cells,[72] also a loss of rhythmic expression of CRY1 and PER2 in fibroblasts.[73] Mice deficient for CRY1 and 2 proteins show an abnormally high level of anxiety.[74] In conclusion, the effects resulting from altered clock genes may play a role in sleep problems and the emergence of symptoms present in certain psychiatric disorders.

Anxiety, stress, and depressive symptoms are often associated with insomnia. Insomnia symptoms are associated with MEIS1 in animal models, it is located near TMEM132E and CYCL1. TMEM132E is a gene family with roles in brain development, panic/anxiety, and bipolar disorder, suggesting a link between insomnia symptoms and an underlying broader sensitivity to anxiety and stress. CYCL1 is a locus previously associated with alcohol dependence comorbid with depressive symptoms.[75]

Symptoms in depression include early morning awakenings and fatigue, these features also indicate disturbed sleep. Neurotransmitters involved in depression are also linked to sleep regulation,

Table 1
Neurodevelopmental syndromes and associated sleep disturbances

Syndromes	SRBD	Insomnia	EDS	Sleep Enuresis	Sleep Bruxism
Angelman	+	+	+	+	+
CHARGE	+	−	-	-	-
Cornelia de Lange	+	+	+	-	-
Cri du Chat	−	−	-	-	-
Down	+	+	+	+	+
Fragile X	+	+	+	+	+
Hurler	+	−	-	-	-
Jacobsen	−	−	-	-	-
Juvenile Neuronal Ceroid Lipofuscinosis	−	−	-	-	-
Mucopolysaccharidoses	+	−	-	-	-
Neurofibromatosis	+	+	+	-	-
Prader-Willi	+	+	+	+	
Rett	+	+	+	-	+
Smith-Magenis	−	+	+	-	-
Smith-Lemli-Opitz	−	−	-	-	-
Tuberous Sclerosis Complex	−	+	+	-	-
Williams	+	+	+	+	+

Abbreviations: EDS, excessive daytime sleepiness; SRBD, sleep-related breathing disorder.
Data from Agar G, Brown C, Sutherland D, Coulborn S, Oliver C, Richards C. Sleep disorders in rare genetic syndromes: a meta-analysis of prevalence and profile. Mol Autism. 2021;12(1):18. https://doi.org/10.1186/s13229-021-00426-w [81]

including serotonergic and glutamatergic neuro-transmission and the hypothalamic-pituitary-adrenal axis. GWA studies from Finland found suggestive associations in women for GAD1, GRIA3, and BDNF with depression accompanied by fatigue, and for CRHR1 with depression accompanied by early morning awakenings.[76]

Almost 80% of schizophrenic patients have sleep disturbance, which are associated with greater symptom severity, increased relapse rates, worse prognoses, and a diminished quality of life.[77] These sleep disturbances may be caused by exogenous effects of psychoactive agents (psychotropic medications, alcohol, illegal substances) or the endogenous effects of disease-related pathophysiological processes on sleep continuity and architecture. Schizophrenic patients report various sleep disorders, mainly insomnia, RLS, and OSA syndrome.[78] Several genetic polymorphisms were associated with schizophrenia-related sleep disorders. Antipsychotic-induced RLS was linked to polymorphisms located on CLOCK (Circadian Locomotor Output Cycles Kaput), BTBD9 (BTB Domain Containing 9), GNB3 (G Protein Subunit Beta 3), and TH (Tyrosine Hydroxylase) genes. Clozapine-induced somnolence was correlated with polymorphisms of HNMT (histamine N-methyltransferase) gene, whereas insomnia symptoms were associated with polymorphisms of the MTNR1 (Melatonin Receptor 1A) gene.[79]

Sleep Disturbance in Neurodevelopmental Disorders

Sleep disturbances are extremely prevalent in children with neurodevelopmental disorders compared with typically developing children. The diagnostic criteria for many neurodevelopmental disorders include sleep disturbances. Sleep disturbance in this population is often multifactorial and caused by the interplay of genetic, neurobiological, and environmental overlap. These disturbances often present either as insomnia or hypersomnia.[80] Insomnia was reported in most syndromes, but it was not associated with specific genetic risk.[81] **Table 1** lists the neurodevelopmental syndromes and their associated sleep disturbances.

SUMMARY

Sleep is a very complex behavior that is influenced by genetic and environmental factors. We still have

Table 2
Genes associated with sleep disorders

Sleep Disorder	Gene
Hypersomnia	
• Narcolepsy	Hypocretin receptor 2 (HCRTR2) or the hypocretin ligand genes (animal models) HLA-DQB1*06:02 gene allele (human) SNP rs5770917 located between CPT1B (carnitine palmitoyltransferase 1B) and CHKB (Choline Kinase B)
• Idiopathic Hypersomnia	HLA-DQB1*06:02 Polymorphism located between CPT1B and CHKB
CRSWD	
• ASWPD	PER2 S662G mutation (in FASPS)
• DSWPD	PER3 and PER3 promoter, CRY1
Restless Legs Syndrome	MEIS1, BTBD9 MAP2K5 and SKOR1(LBXCOR1)
Insomnia	
• Insomnia	MEIS1, CYCL1, TMEM132E, SCFD2
• FNSS	DEC2
SRBD	
• OSA	Angiopoietin-2 gene (ANGPT2), TNF-α gene, prostaglandin E2 receptor (PTGER3) gene, lysophosphatidic acid receptor 1 (LPAR1) gene, G-protein receptor gene (GPR83), β-arrestin 1 (ARRB1) gene
• CCHS	Paired-like homeobox 2B (PHOX2B)
Psychiatric disorder	
• Bipolar disorder	SNP in the 3-flanking region of the Clock gene (3111 T to C), TMEM132 E
• Major depressive disorder	SNPs in the Clock gene (3117 G to T, 3125 A to G), GAD1, GRIA3, BDNF
• Schizophrenia	PER1, PER2, PER3, CRY1, NPAS2, MTNR1 (Melatonin Receptor 1A)
• Anxiety	CRY1, CRY2, TMEM132E
• Alcohol dependence comorbid with depressive symptoms	CYCL1

Abbreviations: ASWPD, advanced sleep-wake phase disorder; CCHS, congenital central hypoventilation syndrome; CRSWD, circadian rhythm sleep-wake disorder; DSWPD, delayed sleep-wake phase disorder; FNSS, familial natural short sleeper; OSA, obstructive sleep apnea; SRDB, sleep-related breathing disorder.

not discovered sleep genes. Many sleep disturbances have underlying genetic factors, but most are caused by the interplay between genetical, environmental, and biological factors. **Table 2** lists sleep disorders and their underlying genetic basis. Some sleep disturbances have polymorphisms in the circadian clock. Moreover, sleep is still an expanding field, there is still a lot more to be discerned. Understanding the genetic factors underlying sleep disturbance may help us to discover the mechanisms of sleep.

CLINICS CARE POINTS

- Recent studies in humans and animal models have uncovered some genetic factors underlying sleep disturbances.
- Sleep is a very complex behavior that is, regulated by circadian rhythm, homeostatic drive, and other processes, all of which have genetic regulation.
- Many sleep disturbances have underlying genetic factors, some caused by polymorphisms of the circadian clock.
- However, most sleep disturbances mechanisms are caused by interaction between genetical, biological and environmental factors.

DISCLOSURE

The author has nothing to disclose.

REFERENCES

1. Sehgal A, Mignot E. Genetics of sleep and sleep disorders. Cell 2011;146(2):194–207.
2. Shi G, Wu D, Ptáček LJ, et al. Human genetics and sleep behavior. Curr Opin Neurobiol 2017;44:43–9.
3. Diessler S, Jan M, Emmenegger Y, et al. A systems genetics resource and analysis of sleep regulation in the mouse. PLoS Biol 2018;16(8):e2005750.
4. Franken P. A role for clock genes in sleep homeostasis. Curr Opin Neurobiol 2013;23(5):864–72.
5. Laposky A, Easton A, Dugovic C, et al. Deletion of the mammalian circadian clock gene BMAL1/Mop3 alters baseline sleep architecture and the response to sleep deprivation. Sleep 2005;28(4):395–409.
6. Zheng X, Sehgal A. Probing the relative importance of molecular oscillations in the circadian clock. Genetics 2008;178(3):1147–55.
7. Cox KH, Takahashi JS. Circadian clock genes and the transcriptional architecture of the clock mechanism. J Mol Endocrinol 2019;63(4):R93–102.
8. Jan M, O'Hara BF, Franken P. Recent advances in understanding the genetics of sleep. F1000Res 2020;9. https://doi.org/10.12688/f1000research.22028.1.
9. Hor CN, Yeung J, Jan M, et al. Sleep–wake-driven and circadian contributions to daily rhythms in gene expression and chromatin accessibility in the murine cortex. Proc Natl Acad Sci U S A 2019;116(51):25773–83.
10. Viola AU, Archer SN, James LM, et al. PER3 polymorphism predicts sleep structure and waking performance. Curr Biol 2007;17(7):613–8.
11. Franken P, Thomason R, Heller HC, et al. A non-circadian role for clock-genes in sleep homeostasis:a strain comparison. BMC Neurosci 2007;8(1):87.
12. Greene RW, Bjorness TE, Suzzuki A. The adenosine-mediated, neuronal-glial, homeostatic sleep response. Curr Opin Neurobiol 2017;44:236–42.
13. Cirelli C, Bushey D, Hill S, et al. Reduced sleep in Drosophila Shaker mutants. Nature 2005;434(7037):1087–92.
14. Imeri L, Opp MR. How (and why) the immune system makes us sleep. Nat Rev Neurosci 2009;10(3):199–210.
15. Asif N, Iqbal R, Nazir CF. Human immune system during sleep. Am J Clin Exp Immunol 2017;6(6):92–6.
16. Chen Z, Gardi J, Kushikata T, et al. Nuclear factor-κB-like activity increases in murine cerebral cortex after sleep deprivation. Am J Physiol 1999;276(6):R1812–8.
17. Williams JA, Sathyanarayanan S, Hendricks JC, et al. Interaction between sleep and the immune response in Drosophila: a role for the NFκB relish. Sleep 2007;30(4):389–400.
18. Ruoff C, Rye D. The ICSD-3 and DSM-5 guidelines for diagnosing narcolepsy: clinical relevance and practicality. Curr Med Res Opin 2016;32(10):1611–22.
19. Lin L, Faraco J, Li R, et al. The sleep disorder canine narcolepsy is caused by a mutation in the hypocretin (orexin) receptor 2 gene. Cell 1999;98(3):365–76.
20. Chemelli RM, Willie JT, Sinton CM, et al. Narcolepsy in orexin knockout mice: molecular genetics of sleep regulation. Cell 1999;98(4):437–51.
21. Miyagawa T, Tokunaga K. Genetics of narcolepsy. Hum Genome Var 2019;6(1):1–8.
22. Mignot E. Genetic and familial aspects of narcolepsy. Neurology 1998;50(2 Suppl 1):S16–22.
23. Sakurai T, Amemiya A, Ishii M, et al. Orexins and orexin receptors: a family of hypothalamic neuropeptides and G protein-coupled receptors that regulate feeding behavior. Cell 1998;92(4):573–85.
24. Sakurai T. The neural circuit of orexin (hypocretin): maintaining sleep and wakefulness. Nat Rev Neurosci 2007;8(3):171–81.
25. Mignot E, Hayduk R, Black J, et al. HLA DQB1*0602 is associated with cataplexy in 509 narcoleptic patients. Sleep 1997;20(11):1012–20.
26. Miyagawa T, Toyoda H, Kanbayashi T, et al. An association analysis of HLA-DQB1 with narcolepsy without cataplexy and idiopathic hypersomnia with/without long sleep time in a Japanese population. Hum Genome Variation 2015;2(1):1–4.

27. Mignot E, Lin L, Rogers W, et al. Complex HLA-DR and -DQ interactions confer risk of narcolepsy-cataplexy in three ethnic groups. Am J Hum Genet 2001;68(3):686–99.

28. Han F, Lin L, Warby SC, et al. Narcolepsy onset is seasonal and increased following the 2009 H1N1 pandemic in China. Ann Neurol 2011;70(3):410–7.

29. Nohynek H, Jokinen J, Partinen M, et al. AS03 adjuvanted AH1N1 vaccine associated with an abrupt increase in the incidence of childhood narcolepsy in Finland. PLoS One 2012;7(3):e33536.

30. Dauvilliers Y, Arnulf I, Lecendreux M, et al. Increased risk of narcolepsy in children and adults after pandemic H1N1 vaccination in France. Brain 2013;136(8):2486–96.

31. Miyagawa T, Kawashima M, Nishida N, et al. Variant between CPT1B and CHKB associated with susceptibility to narcolepsy. Nat Genet 2008;40(11):1324–8.

32. Miyagawa T, Honda M, Kawashima M, et al. Polymorphism located between CPT1B and CHKB, and HLA-DRB1*1501-DQB1*0602 haplotype confer susceptibility to CNS hypersomnias (essential hypersomnia). PLOS ONE 2009;4(4):e5394.

33.. American Academy of Sleep Medicine. International classification of sleep disorders. 3rd edition. Darien (IL): American Academy of Sleep Medicine; 2014.

34. Curtis BJ, Ashbrook LH, Young T, et al. Extreme morning chronotypes are often familial and not exceedingly rare: the estimated prevalence of advanced sleep phase, familial advanced sleep phase, and advanced sleep–wake phase disorder in a sleep clinic population. Sleep 2019;42(10):zsz148.

35. Toh KL, Jones CR, He Y, et al. An hPer2 phosphorylation site mutation in familial advanced sleep phase syndrome. Science 2001;291(5506):1040–3.

36. Xu Y, Padiath QS, Shapiro RE, et al. Functional consequences of a CKIδ mutation causing familial advanced sleep phase syndrome. Nature 2005; 434(7033):640–4.

37. Xu Y, Toh KL, Jones CR, et al. Modeling of a human circadian mutation yields insights into clock regulation by PER2. Cell 2007;128(1):59–70.

38. Jones CR, Huang AL, Ptáček LJ, et al. Genetic basis of human circadian rhythm disorders. Exp Neurol 2013;243:28–33.

39. Archer SN, Robilliard DL, Skene DJ, et al. A length polymorphism in the circadian clock gene Per3 is linked to delayed sleep phase syndrome and extreme diurnal preference. Sleep 2003;26(4): 413–5.

40. Archer SN, Carpen JD, Gibson M, et al. Polymorphism in the PER3 promoter associates with diurnal preference and delayed sleep phase disorder. Sleep 2010;33(5):695–701.

41. Osland TM, Bjorvatn BR, Steen VM, et al. Association study of a variable-number tandem repeat polymorphism in the clock gene PERIOD3 and chronotype in Norwegian university students. Chronobiol Int 2011;28(9):764–70.

42. Patke A, Murphy PJ, Onat OE, et al. Mutation of the human circadian clock gene CRY1 in familial delayed sleep phase disorder. Cell 2017;169(2): 203–15.e13.

43. Salas RE, Gamaldo CE, Allen RP. Update in restless legs syndrome. Curr Opin Neurol 2010;23(4):401–6.

44. Gonzalez-Latapi P, Malkani R. Update on restless legs syndrome: from mechanisms to treatment. Curr Neurol Neurosci Rep 2019;19(8):54.

45. Winkelmann J, Schormair B, Lichtner P, et al. Genome-wide association study of restless legs syndrome identifies common variants in three genomic regions. Nat Genet 2007;39(8):1000–6.

46. Lyu S, Xing H, DeAndrade MP, et al. The Role of BTBD9 in Striatum and Restless Legs Syndrome. eNeuro 2019;6(5). ENEURO.0277-19.2019.

47. Rizzo G, Li X, Galantucci S, et al. Brain imaging and networks in restless legs syndrome. Sleep Med 2017;31:39–48.

48. Earley CJ, Kuwabara H, Wong DF, et al. The dopamine transporter is decreased in the striatum of subjects with restless legs syndrome. Sleep 2011;34(3):341–7.

49. Michaud M, Soucy J-P, Chabli A, et al. SPECT imaging of striatal pre- and postsynaptic dopaminergic status in restless legs syndrome with periodic leg movements in sleep. J Neurol 2002;249(2):164–70.

50. Stefansson H, Rye DB, Hicks A, et al. A genetic risk factor for periodic limb movements in sleep. N Engl J Med 2007;357(7):639–47.

51. Lane JM, Jones SE, Dashti HS, et al. Biological and clinical insights from genetics of insomnia symptoms. Nat Genet 2019;51(3):387–93.

52. Llorens F, Zarranz J-J, Fischer A, et al. Fatal familial insomnia: clinical aspects and molecular alterations. Curr Neurol Neurosci Rep 2017;17(4):30.

53. Medori R, Tritschler HJ, LeBlanc A, et al. Fatal familial insomnia, a prion disease with a mutation at codon 178 of the prion protein gene. N Engl J Med 1992;326(7):444–9.

54. Cortelli P, Gambetti P, Montagna P, et al. Fatal familial insomnia: clinical features and molecular genetics. J Sleep Res 1999;8(Suppl 1):23–9.

55. He Y, Jones CR, Fujiki N, et al. The transcriptional repressor DEC2 regulates sleep length in mammals. Science 2009;325(5942):866–70.

56. Honma S, Kawamoto T, Takagi Y, et al. Dec1 and Dec2 are regulators of the mammalian molecular clock. Nature 2002;419(6909):841–4.

57. Hirano A, Hsu P-K, Zhang L, et al. DEC2 modulates orexin expression and regulates sleep. Proc Natl Acad Sci U S A 2018;115(13):3434–9.

58. Tanizawa K, Chin K. Genetic factors in sleep-disordered breathing. Respir Investig 2018;56(2): 111–9.

59. Redline S, Tosteson T, Tishler PV, et al. Studies in the genetics of obstructive sleep apnea. Familial aggregation of symptoms associated with sleep-related breathing disturbances. Am Rev Respir Dis 1992; 145(2 Pt 1):440–4.

60. Mukherjee S, Saxena R, Palmer LJ. The genetics of obstructive sleep apnoea. Respirology 2018;23(1): 18–27.

61. Redline S, Tishler PV. The genetics of sleep apnea. Sleep Med Rev 2000;4(6):583–602.

62. Patel SR, Frame JM, Larkin EK, et al. Heritability of upper airway dimensions derived using acoustic pharyngometry. Eur Respir J 2008;32(5):1304–8.

63. Herrera BM, Lindgren CM. The genetics of obesity. Curr Diab Rep 2010;10(6):498–505.

64. Roosenboom J, Hens G, Mattern BC, et al. Exploring the underlying genetics of craniofacial morphology through various sources of knowledge. Biomed Res Int 2016;2016:3054578.

65. Weil JV. Variation in human ventilatory control—genetic influence on the hypoxic ventilatory response. Respir Physiol Neurobiol 2003;135(2):239–46.

66. Wang H, Cade BE, Chen H, et al. Variants in angiopoietin-2 (ANGPT2) contribute to variation in nocturnal oxyhaemoglobin saturation level. Hum Mol Genet 2016;25(23):5244–53.

67. Bhushan B, Guleria R, Misra A, et al. TNF-alpha gene polymorphism and TNF-alpha levels in obese Asian Indians with obstructive sleep apnea. Respir Med 2009;103(3):386–92.

68. Amiel J, Laudier B, Attié-Bitach T, et al. Polyalanine expansion and frameshift mutations of the paired-like homeobox gene PHOX2B in congenital central hypoventilation syndrome. Nat Genet 2003;33(4): 459–61.

69. Weese-Mayer DE, Berry-Kravis EM, Ceccherini I, et al. An official ATS clinical policy statement: congenital central hypoventilation syndrome. Am J Respir Crit Care Med 2010;181(6):626–44.

70. Charrier A, Olliac B, Roubertoux P, et al. Clock genes and altered sleep–wake rhythms: their role in the development of psychiatric disorders. Int J Mol Sci 2017;18(5):938.

71. Benedetti F, Dallaspezia S, Fulgosi MC, et al. Actimetric evidence that CLOCK 3111 T/C SNP influences sleep and activity patterns in patients affected by bipolar depression. Am J Med Genet B Neuropsychiatr Genet 2007;144B(5):631–5.

72. Sun H-Q, Li S-X, Chen F-B, et al. Diurnal neurobiological alterations after exposure to clozapine in first-episode schizophrenia patients. Psychoneuroendocrinology 2016;64:108–16.

73. Johansson A-S, Owe-Larsson B, Hetta J, et al. Altered circadian clock gene expression in patients with schizophrenia. Schizophr Res 2016;174(1–3): 17–23.

74. De Bundel D, Gangarossa G, Biever A, et al. Cognitive dysfunction, elevated anxiety, and reduced cocaine response in circadian clock-deficient cryptochrome knockout mice. Front Behav Neurosci 2013;7. https://doi.org/10.3389/fnbeh.2013.00152.

75. Lane JM, Liang J, Vlasac I, et al. Genome-wide association analyses of sleep disturbance traits identify new loci and highlight shared genetics with neuropsychiatric and metabolic traits. Nat Genet 2017;49(2):274–81.

76. Utge S, Soronen P, Partonen T, et al. A population-based association study of candidate genes for depression and sleep disturbance. Am J Med Genet B Neuropsychiatr Genet 2010;153B(2):468–76.

77. Afonso P, Brissos S, Figueira ML, et al. Schizophrenia patients with predominantly positive symptoms have more disturbed sleep-wake cycles measured by actigraphy. Psychiatry Res 2011; 189(1):62–6.

78. Kaskie RE, Graziano B, Ferrarelli F. Schizophrenia and sleep disorders: links, risks, and management challenges. Nat Sci Sleep 2017;9:227–39.

79. Assimakopoulos K, Karaivazoglou K, Skokou M, et al. Genetic variations associated with sleep disorders in patients with schizophrenia: a systematic review. Medicines (Basel) 2018;5(2):27.

80. Robinson-Shelton A, Malow BA. Sleep disturbances in neurodevelopmental disorders. Curr Psychiatry Rep 2015;18(1):6.

81. Agar G, Brown C, Sutherland D, et al. Sleep disorders in rare genetic syndromes: a meta-analysis of prevalence and profile. Mol Autism 2021;12(1):18.

Abnormal Sleep-Related Breathing Related to Heart Failure

Tripat Deep Singh, MBBS, MD, RPSGT, RST

KEYWORDS

- Sleep-disordered breathing • Heart failure • Positive airway pressure • Obstructive sleep apnea
- Central sleep apnea • Cheyne Stokes breathing

KEY POINTS

- Heart failure (HF) is leading comorbidity for hospitalization in United States
- Sleep-disordered breathing (SDB) is highly prevalent in patients with HF
- SDB should be routinely screened in patients with HF with routine clinical history
- Obstructive sleep apnea (OSA) in HF can be effectively treated with continuous positive airway pressure (CPAP) therapy with consistent reports of improvement in left ventricular ejection fraction
- There is a lack of evidence to suggest any effective therapy for treating central sleep apnea (CSA) in patients with HF

INTRODUCTION

Heart failure (HF) is a major medical problem affecting 26 million people worldwide.[1] HF is the most frequent cause of hospitalization in the United States Medicare system accounting for 1%–2% of all hospitalizations.[2] HF and other comorbidities leading to HF needs to be identified and treated early as the total costs of HF management are estimated to increase from $31 billion in 2012 to $70 billion in 2030 in the US only.[3] Sleep-disordered breathing (SDB) is one comorbidity which is under-recognized but highly prevalent in both systolic and diastolic HF, affecting 50% to 80% of all patients with HF.[4–6] SDB is classified further into obstructive sleep apnea (OSA) and central sleep apnea (CSA). Both OSA and CSA lead to repetitive hypoxemia and arousals leading to sympathetic excitation, oxidative/nitrosative stress, and sleep disruption leading to a negative impact on patients with HF.

In this article, we will discuss the known science of how different SDB affects HF and how to manage different SDB in patients with HF.

EPIDEMIOLOGY OF SLEEP-DISORDERED BREATHING HEART FAILURE

HF can be described as systolic versus diastolic, heart failure with preserved ejection fraction (HFpEF) versus heart failure with reduced ejection fraction (HFrEF), acute versus chronic HF, and right-sided versus left-sided HF. SDB is highly prevalent in all types of HF.

Sixty-six percent (66%) of individuals with asymptomatic left ventricular systolic dysfunction experienced moderate-to-severe sleep apnea: 55% with CSA and 11% with OSA.[7] Presence of undiagnosed OSA and CSA in asymptomatic left ventricular dysfunction can lead to progression from asymptomatic to symptomatic condition.[8–10]

Prevalence of OSA is less studied in diastolic HF. One study reported a 50% prevalence of OSA (Apnea Hypopnea Index [AHI]>10/h) in isolated diastolic HF.[11]

Fifty-three (53%) of 1607 patients with HFrEF had moderate-to-severe sleep apnea (defined as an AHI ≥15): 34% had CSA and 19% had OSA.[12]

The prevalence of sleep apnea in HFpEF is similar to that in HFrEF. Combining 2 studies

Academy of Sleep Wake Science, #32 St.no-9 Guru Nanak Nagar, near Gurbax Colony, Patiala, Punjab, India 147003
E-mail address: tripatdeepsingh@gmail.com

Sleep Med Clin 17 (2022) 87–98
https://doi.org/10.1016/j.jsmc.2021.10.007
1556-407X/22/© 2021 Elsevier Inc. All rights reserved.

(79,80) with a total of 263 consecutive patients, 47% had sleep apnea (AHI $\geq$15): 24% OSA and 23% CSA.[12]

With fall in ejection fraction (EF), the prevalence of SDB increases considerably in HF. In 1117 patients with consecutive HFrEF hospitalized with acute HF who underwent in-hospital polysomnography, 31% had CSA and 47% had OSA.[13]

Patients with HF can shift from one SDB type to another on a night to night basis.[14] Patients with HF with OSA can have a significant number of central events but prevalence of such cases is not well studied. Both types of SDB can be seen together in the same patient with HF.

PATHOPHYSIOLOGY OF OBSTRUCTIVE SLEEP APNEA IN HEART FAILURE

Anatomic (narrow upper airway) and nonanatomical (high loop gain, low arousal threshold, reduced pharyngeal dilator muscle tone, and fluid shift) factors have been recognized as underlying causes of OSA.[15] Identifying the underlying cause in each OSA patient and starting appropriate therapy forms the basis of personalized medicine for OSA. Loop gain, low arousal threshold, and reduced pharyngeal dilator muscle tone have been studied in detail in OSA patients without HF.

Repetitive closure of upper airway in patients with OSA leads to cyclic intermittent hypoxia which causes sympathetic excitation[16] leading to pulmonary and systemic vasoconstriction.[17] Intermittent hypoxia also causes daytime hypertension[18,19] and is an independent risk factor for hypertension[20] and ischemic heart disease.[21,22] Increased sympathetic activation also increases the heart rate which increases the myocardial metabolic requirement leading to ischemia, myocyte irritability, and arrhythmias.[23] OSA is also associated with known risk factors for HF such as coronary artery disease,[24] hypertension, and arrhythmias.[25]

During an apneic event, upper airway is occluded but there is continuous effort to breathe. This results in negative intrathoracic pressure which increases left ventricular transmural gradient thereby increasing afterload and decreasing cardiac output.[26] Negative intrathoracic pressure also increases venous return to the right ventricle. This increased venous return overfills the right ventricle which causes the interventricular septum to bulge toward left decreasing the left ventricular volume and hence cardiac output, leading to poor circulation.[27]

Due to all the above factors, OSA can lead to the development of new HF in patients with untreated OSA. OSA predicted incident HF in men but not in women (adjusted hazard ratio 1.13 [95% confidence interval (CI): 1.02–1.26] per 10-unit increase in AHI). Men with AHI > or = 30 were 58% more likely to develop HF than those with AHI less than 5.[9]

Obesity contributes less to OSA in patients with HF than patients without HF.[28] In patients with nonobese HF, central and cranial fluid shifts happening in supine position cause neck congestion, pharyngeal edema, and upper airway obstruction.[29,30]

PATHOPHYSIOLOGY OF CENTRAL SLEEP APNEA IN HEART FAILURE

The most common type of CSA seen in patients with HF is Cheyne-Stokes Respiration (CSR). Normal spontaneous respiration is regulated by levels of CO_2 in blood via chemoreceptors. In CSR, chemoreceptors become hypersensitive to CO_2 (high loop gain) leading to hyperventilation, which brings CO_2 levels below the apneic threshold and apnea occurs.

Pulmonary congestion seen in HF also causes hyperventilation by stimulating stretch receptors in lung leading to CO_2 levels to fall below apneic threshold and loss of respiratory drive.[31]

Other factors that cause cyclic CSA events are upper airway instability, diminished cerebrovascular response to changes in Pa_{CO_2} levels, low cardiac output with resultant prolonged circulation, and mismatch between central and peripheral chemoreceptor responses.[32–35]

Cyclical CSA events lead to harmful hemodynamic changes like tachycardia, systemic vasoconstriction, activation of renin–angiotensin system, and fluid retention deleterious to heart function.[36,37] CSA also leads to sympathetic excitation predisposing to arrhythmias and this risk can be decreased by treating CSA.[38,39] CSA presence in patients with HF is associated with worse prognosis leading to more hospital admissions, cardiac transplantation, and death.[40,41]

EVALUATION OF SLEEP-DISORDERED BREATHING IN HEART FAILURE

A comprehensive sleep history should be taken in all HF in and out patients. A high level of suspicion should be maintained for SDB in patients with HF due to atypical presentation of SDB in patients with HF.

For OSA, the examiner should focus on the presence of male sex, older age, obesity, and history of snoring. However, sleepiness, a classical presentation of SDB, is less seen in patients with HF.[28,42] Questionnaires such as Epworth

Sleepiness Scale (ESS) have been found to be less effective in screening for OSA in patients with HF.[28] Also, obesity contributes less to OSA in patients with HF than patients without HF.[28] Data regarding the Mallampati airway classification to assess the severity of upper airway obstruction are lacking in patients with HF.

Clinical assessment for CSA is more difficult. For CSA, the examiner should look for advanced HF, low functional class, low left ventricular ejection fraction (LVEF), high brain natriuretic peptide (BNP) levels, and nocturnal ventricular tachycardia (VT).[4,43–45]

If there is a high suspicion of SDB on clinical history and examination, nocturnal polysomnography (PSG) is currently recommended for diagnosing SDB in patients with HF. AASM recommends that polysomnography, rather than home sleep apnea testing (HST), should be used for the diagnosis of OSA in patients with significant cardiorespiratory disease.[46] Although, a recent study has shown that HST can help to diagnose SDB and identify OSA, CSA, and Cheyne-Stokes Respiration (CSR) events in adults with HF.[47]

TREATMENT OF OBSTRUCTIVE SLEEP APNEA IN HEART FAILURE

First step in the management of HF with OSA is restoring euvolemia with diuretics, optimizing/starting guideline-directed medical therapy (GDMT), or cardiac resynchronization therapy.

Positive airway pressure (PAP) therapy

PAP devices including CPAP and Bilevel PAP are the most effective form of treatment of OSA in the general population and in patients with HF. AASM has been recommended to treat patients with OSA with excessive daytime sleepiness (EDS), hypertension, or poor quality of life with PAP therapy.[48] PAP therapy to treat OSA in patients with HF should be started after optimizing GDMT and high suspicion of underlying OSA is present.

PAP therapy has several beneficial effects in patients with decompensated HF and pulmonary edema—improves gas exchange, increases LVEF, and reduces left ventricular filling pressure.[49] In patients with HF with OSA, CPAP therapy has been shown to reduce myocardial muscle energy consumption.[50] In patients with HF, treatment with CPAP reduced respiratory and cardiac muscle workload.[51] One study also showed that treatment with CPAP reduced hospitalizations and improved mortality in HF patients with OSA.[52] In patients with hospitalized decompensated HF with OSA, treatment with CPAP

improved the LVEF after discharge.[53] In patients with stable HF with OSA, treatment with CPAP improved sympathetic overactivity,[54,55] cardiac vagal tone,[56] and cardiac afterload.[57]

The beneficial effects of PAP therapy in patients with HF are due to an increase in the intrathoracic pressure which decreases transmural cardiac pressure reducing myocardium workload and oxygen consumption.[58,59] One should be careful in right-sided HF whereby the right ventricle is preload dependent as increased intrathoracic pressure may decrease venous return to the right ventricle and increase right ventricle afterload by increasing the lung volume. These changes can be deleterious to the failing right ventricle. Other mechanisms contributing to beneficial effects of CPAP on heart function in patients with HF are-[60]

1. Reduction in intrathoracic pressure swings by the elimination of apneas and hypopneas reduces work of breathing and improves oxygenation
2. CPAP therapy shifts the interstitial fluid into vascular compartment which improves ventilation-perfusion mismatches thereby improving oxygenation
3. Reduced stimulation of intrapulmonary vagal afferents which dampens ventilatory overshoot and stabilizes the breathing

All these results looked promising in treating OSA in patients with HF with CPAP. But a recent RCT (SAVE trial) showed that the treatment of patients with OSA with existing coronary or cerebrovascular disease does not prevent future cardiovascular events.[61] SAVE trial was an international multicentre RCT which included 2717 moderate to severe patients with non-sleepy OSA with existing coronary or cerebrovascular disease. The patients were followed up for 3.7 years. The major limitations of the SAVE trial which might have affected the unexpected results of the trial were the inclusion of patients with non-sleepy OSA, low CPAP adherence (3.3 hr/night), and exclusion of patients with HF in NYHA functional class III and IV.[62] SAVE trial showed improvement in quality of life and daytime sleepiness in patients with OSA treated with CPAP. The results of the SAVE trial suggest that CPAP can be used to treat patients with OSA with existing coronary or cerebrovascular disease to improve their quality of life and daytime sleepiness but not to prevent future cardiovascular events. SAVE study also does not offer any insights into the efficacy of CPAP in the primary prevention of cardiovascular outcomes in patients with OSA.[60]

Treating high loop gain

It has been shown that high loop gain contributes to the severity of OSA.[63] There is debate about whether high loop gain in OSA is due to genetic predisposition or is the consequence of severe OSA. In a recent review, authors concluded that irrespective of the time course as to when loop gain was acquired, it may contribute to worsening of OSA and may be a potential therapeutic target.[64]

Two medications, oxygen[65,66] and acetazol-amide[67,68] have been used to treat OSA in patients without HF. But it needs to be studied whether oxygen, acetazolamide, or their combination can be used to treat OSA in patients with HF with elevated loop gain. This can be a potential treatment given the poor adherence to CPAP therapy in patients with OSA.

Treating low arousal threshold

Trazodone[69] and eszopiclone[70] have been used in treating OSA in patients without HF with limited success. Authors in a recent review have raised concerns regarding using drugs to prolong arousal traits to treat OSA in patients with cardiovascular disorders including HF.[64]

Oral appliances

Oral appliances have been used to treat OSA in patients with HF without estimating anatomic compromise. Studies have shown that some patients with OSA with HF respond, and some do not respond to oral appliance therapy.[71,72] A large trial in patients with HF with OSA and anatomically narrow airway is warranted for more suggestions on this therapy.

Upper airway stimulation

It has been used to treat OSA in general population, in patients with PAP intolerance , or who refuse PAP therapy. Trials in patients with HF with OSA are still awaited. Authors in a recent review have suggested choosing patients with OSA with HF very carefully for this therapy given the risk of anesthesia and implantation in patients with HF.[64]

Exercise and obstructive sleep apnea in heart failure

In HFrEF, both exercise and CPAP improved subjective daytime sleepiness, quality of life, and New York Heart Association (NYHA) functional class.[73] Exercise alone led to a 35% reduction in AHI[73] similar to another study.[74] In patients with HF, exercise and cardiac rehabilitation decrease exertional oscillatory ventilation.[73,75] The beneficial effects of exercise may be mediated via weight loss, decrease in lower extremity edema,[29] down-regulation of hypercapnic ventilatory response attenuating loop gain.[76] Oropharyngeal exercises are also useful in maintaining upper airway patency by exerting a local effect.[77]

TREATMENT OF CENTRAL SLEEP APNEA IN HEART FAILURE

First step in the management of HF with CSA is restoring euvolemia with diuretics, optimizing/starting guideline-directed medical therapy (GDMT) or cardiac resynchronization therapy and cardiac transplantation. GDMT improves CSA in patients with HF by improving circulation time by increasing stroke volume and cardiac output.[78] Cardiac transplantation is the most effective treatment for HFrEF having CSA although there was unexplained development of restless legs syndrome and periodic limb movements.[79]

Non-positive airway pressure therapies

A. Therapies targeting loop gain
1. Low flow nocturnal oxygen therapy (NOXT)

In patients with HFrEF and CSA, there is sympathetic overexcitation in muscle[80] and heart,[81] and high morning plasma and overnight urinary catecholamines[82] mediated by peripheral and central chemoreceptors hypersensitivity to hypoxia and hypercapnia which is associated with worse prognosis.[83] Thus, decreasing carotid body hyper-response to hypoxia with oxygen therapy becomes an important therapeutic target to treat CSA in patients with HF.

NOXT have been shown to attenuate CSA/CSB[84] but with variable response.[85] NOXT abolishes desaturations[85] which may have survival benefit as oxygen desaturation index (ODI) has been shown to be a predictor of mortality in patients with HFrEF who were followed up for 10 yrs.[86]

NOXT improves outcomes in patients with HFrEF with CSA by decreasing the sympathetic activity[87,88] and improves the quality of life (QOL) after 3 months.[89,90] These results are encouraging and raise the hope that NOXT may improve the mortality in patients with HFrEF with CSA. Recently National Institute of Health (NIH) have funded a trial to evaluate the effect of oxygen versus GDMT care in patients with HFrEF with CSA: The Impact of Low Flow Oxygen Therapy on Hospital Admissions and Mortality in Patients with Heart Failure and Central Sleep Apnea - Low flow oxygen therapy in heart failure (LOFT-HF) Study (Clinical trials # CT03745898). The primary outcome is the first occurrence of a composite endpoint of mortality, a life-saving cardiovascular (CV) intervention, or unplanned hospitalization for worsening HF.

In patients with normoxic chronic HF, home oxygen therapy given mainly during daytime did not decrease disease severity or improve QOL.[91] Also, oxygen toxicity has been reported in patients with normoxic HF with CSA when oxygen was administered during daytime.[92–94] These studies make the results of LOFT-HF trial highly awaited.

2. Acetazolamide and theophylline

Acetazolamide improves CSA in patients with HFrEF by increasing the difference between existing $Paco_2$ and apneic threshold $Paco_2$,[95] mild diuretic effect[96] and correcting alkalemia[97] prevalent in patients with HF.

Theophylline treatment has shown responders and nonresponders in patients with HFrEF with CSA.[98]

3. Carotid body ablation or denervation

Animal studies of HF have confirmed that the ablation of carotid body abolishes CSA and improves survival.[99,100] Limited human data have shown a reduction in AHI but worsening of other respiratory PSG parameters.[101,102]

B. Treatment of low arousal threshold

Like OSA in HF, there is limited inconclusive data regarding targeting a low arousal threshold for treating CSA in patients with HF. One trial used temazepam showed no improvement in CSA/CSB.[103]

C. Oral appliances for the treatment of CSA in patients with HF

In some CSA with patients with HF, upper airway may close during CSA events.[104] Custom made oral appliances and tongue retaining devices have been used for the treatment of CSA in poorly characterized patients with HF.[105] Treatment-emergent CSA has been reported with the use of mandibular advancement device used for treating OSA.[106] There is not much conclusive data to recommend regular use of oral appliances for treating CSA in patients with HF.

Positive airway pressure therapy

CPAP, BiPAP s/T, and BiPAP ASV have been used to treat CSA in patients with HF.

A. Continuous positive airway pressure for treating central sleep apnea in patients with HF

In some CSA with HF patients, the upper airway may close during CSA events.[104] CPAP may improve cardiac function owing to improved oxygenation and other mechanical factors as discussed earlier. CPAP treatment has been shown to improve LVEF[49,53] but it has not translated into improved mortality in large clinical trials. Canadian continuous positive airway pressure (CanPAP) trial showed improvement in the number of apneas and hypopneas, oxygen saturation, ejection fraction, norepinephrine levels, and exercise performance after treatment with CPAP in patients with HF but no survival benefit.[107] In a post hoc analysis of CanPAP trial data, better survival was reported in responders versus non-responders to CPAP treatment.[108] In patients with HF with CSA, high loop gain has been shown to be associated with poor response to CPAP.[109]

There is insufficient evidence to recommend auto CPAP or BiPAP to treat CSA/CSB in patients with HF.

B. Adaptive servo-ventilation for treating central sleep apnea in patients with heart failure

This PAP technology was developed to treat Cheyne-Stokes breathing (CSB) seen in congestive patients with HF or sometimes in patients with stroke. CSB has a crescendo-decrescendo breathing pattern with central hypopnea or apnea. The theory behind ASV is that it acts to counterbalance this pattern of CSB by varying the pressure support out of sync with patient's own respiration, thereby dampening the factors leading to CSB. It also splints the upper airway by applying fixed or variable EPAP just like BiPAP to treat obstructive apneas. It also delivers mandatory breaths in a timed back-up mode to treat central apneas. These multiple approaches to treat CSB, obstructive, and central apneas make ASV an ideal device to treat patients having both obstructive and central events. There are currently 3 manufacturers for ASV devices and each has a different operational algorithm. The details about each manufacturer ASV device algorithm have been summarized in a recent review article.[110]

In 2012, AASM published guidelines for treating CSA in which they suggested ASV as first-line therapy for treating Central Sleep Apnea Syndrome (CSAS) in patients with HF.[111] In 2015, SERVE-HF study[112] reported that in patients with

HF with reduced ejection fraction and predominantly CSA, treatment with ASV led to an increase in all cause and cardiovascular mortality. As a result, an emergency notice was issued worldwide and many patients who were using ASV were called back to the clinics and informed about the findings of the study and many were taken off ASV therapy. In light of these findings, AASM revised their guidelines for treating CSAS in patients with HF.[113] They recommended that ASV should not be used to treat CSAS in patients with HF with ejection fraction less than 45% and moderate to severe CSAS. Though an option was given to use ASV to treat CSAS in patients with HF with ejection fraction greater than 45% or mild HF-related CSAS.[113] The authors emphasized that SERVE-HF results cannot be extrapolated to patients with HFrEF with OSA because OSA causes more adverse cardiac loading than CSA, which are reversible by positive airway pressure devices.[112]

SERVE-HF study did not explain the cause of increased mortality in patients with HF with reduced ejection fraction and moderate to severe CSAS by using ASV. In a recently published major preplanned sub-study of SERVE-HF,[114] in patients with systolic HF and CSA, addition of ASV to guideline-based medical management had no statistically significant effect on cardiac structure and function, or on cardiac biomarkers, renal function, and systemic inflammation over 12 months. Authors suggested the increased cardiovascular mortality reported in SERVE-HF may not be related to adverse remodeling or worsening HF.[114]

A flurry of editorials and comments were published on the SERVE-HF study challenging the study design and methodology for the results.[115–118] One of the limitations identified was the intention to treat analysis used to analyze the results, and it was suggested that an on-treatment analysis was a better way to analyze the outcome. However, a recent publication on SERVE-HF reported that an on-treatment analysis showed similar results to the SERVE-HF intention-to-treat analysis, with an increased risk of cardiovascular death in patients with HFrEF with predominant CSA treated with adaptive servo-ventilation.[119]

Only one manufacturer's (RESMED) device was used in the SERVE-HF study, so it is not clear whether the results could be influenced by the device's algorithm.[112] To know whether the results were influenced by device-specific algorithm, authors of the SERVE-HF trial suggested to wait for the results of an ongoing trial called Adaptive Servo Ventilation (ASV) on Survival and Hospital Admissions in Heart Failure (ADVENT-HF).[112,120]

ADVENT-HF is designed to assess the effects of treating SDB with ASV on morbidity and mortality in patients with HF[120] and reduced ejection fraction but it is different from the SERVE-HF trial in several respects.[118] It also includes patients with non-sleepy OSA and uses a device from another manufacturer (Philips Respironics) and most of the patients are using a nasal mask with ASV unlike SERVE-HF whereby most of the patients used oro-nasal mask.[118] At the time of writing this article, the results of the ADVENT-HF trial were awaited eagerly by the medical community and patients alike.

Studies published after the SERVE-HF trial do not report similar findings to the SERVE-HF study. After discontinuation of ASV in HF with CSR patient's (LVEF<45%) for 3 months, quality of life (QOL) decreased significantly.[121] Though there was no significant change in NYHA functional class, patients especially reported increased shortness of breath, reduced concentration, and reduced memory after the discontinuation of ASV treatment. There were no significant differences in LVEF, heart rhythm data, and physical capacity. Left ventricular function was preserved indicating that the discontinuation of ASV in patients with HF does not affect cardiac capacity. There was a significant decrement in QOL and authors suggest that QOL must be considered in further treatment of these patients. Median machine use was 68 (42–78) months when the patients were instructed to terminate ASV treatment.[121]

In an RCT, the use of adaptive servo-ventilation improved the quality of life in patients with chronic HF with Cheyne-Stokes respiration. Fifty-one patients (ranging from 53 to 84 years), New York Heart Association III-IV and/or left ventricular ejection fraction ≤40% and Cheyne-Stokes respiration were included in the study.[122]

Another study reported that ASV therapy reduces hospital admissions in patients with severe CHF who are receiving maximum medical treatment.[123] Hospitalization frequencies during the 12 months before and 12 months after the initiation of ASV therapy (24 consecutive months) were retrospectively compared in 44 consecutive patients with severe CHF. The admission frequency decreased from 1.9 ± 1.4 admissions in the 12 months before ASV to 1.1 ± 1.6 admissions in the 12 months after ASV initiation ($P < .001$). The decrease tended to be greater in those patients with more frequent hospitalizations before ASV initiation.[123] A more recent study also reported decreased hospitalization in patients with CHF treated with ASV but also decreased medical costs over 1-year period.[124]

At present, ASV should not be used to treat CSAS in patients with HF with ejection fraction less than 45% and moderate to severe CSAS.

OTHER THERAPIES
Transvenous phrenic nerve stimulation

The major muscle of respiration is the diaphragm which is innervated by the phrenic nerve. In CSA, the patient's brain does not send signals to the respiratory system and so the patient suffers from apnea, desaturations, and arousals. Unlike OSA, treatment of CSA with various PAP modalities has resulted in variable response as highlighted in the ASV section. Phrenic nerve stimulation is a new way to physiologically initiate respiration. Currently, phrenic nerve stimulation is used as therapy in patients with Ondine's curse or high cervical spinal cord injury.[125,126] The current method of transthoracic placement of electrodes to stimulate phrenic nerve may result in complications[127] but a transvenous route is considered to be safer.

A new system, called Remede system, has been developed to stimulate phrenic nerve transvenously.[128] In this study, unilateral stimulation of phrenic nerve led to the reduction of CSA and restoration of normal breathing pattern in patients with HF.[128] There is an ongoing RCT to check the safety and efficacy of Remede system in treating CSA in patients with HF.[129] In a recent nonrandomized study of Remede system over a period of 12 months, treatment of CSA with this system led to significant improvement in sleep parameters, sleep symptoms, and quality of life.[130] Other nonrandomized trials also have shown that the chronic use of phrenic nerve stimulation is safe and feasible in treating CSA in patients with HF.[131]

However, its long-term effects on mortality and morbidity in HFrEF remain to be evaluated.

SUMMARY

SDB is highly prevalent in patients with HF. Untreated OSA and CSA in patients with HF are associated with worse outcomes. Detailed sleep history along with PSG should be conducted if SDB is suspected in patients with HF. First line of treatment is the optimization of medical therapy for HF and if symptoms persist despite optimization of the treatment, start PAP therapy to treat SDB. At present, there is limited evidence to prescribe any drugs for treating CSA in patients with HF. There is limited evidence for the efficacy of CPAP or ASV in improving mortality in patients with HFrEF. There is a need to perform well-designed studies to identify different phenotypes of CSA/OSA in patients with HF and to determine which phenotype responds to which therapy. Results of ongoing trials, ADVENT-HF and LOFT-HF, are eagerly awaited to shed more light on the management of CSA in patients with HF. Until then, management of SDB in patients with HF is limited due to the lack of evidence and guidance for treating SDB in patients with HF.

CLINICS CARE POINTS

- First step in the management of HF with OSA is restoring euvolemia with diuretics, optimizing/starting guideline-directed medical therapy (GDMT), or cardiac resynchronization therapy.
- PAP therapy for treatment of OSA in HF patients lead to improvement in Left ventricular ejection fraction.
- CSA-CSB in HF patients with ejection fraction >45% can be treated with CPAP or ASV.
- ASV is contraindicated for treating CSA-CSB in HF patients with ejection fraction <45%.

CONFLICT OF INTEREST

T. Deep Singh is a Chief Medical Officer for REM42. This work has been compiled by T. Deep Singh and his association with REM42 has not influenced his writing in any way.

REFERENCES

1. Ambrosy AP, Fonarow GC, Butler J, et al. The global health and economic burden of hospitalizations for heart failure: lessons learned from hospitalized heart failure registries. J Am Coll Cardiol 2014;63(12):1123–33.
2. Blecker S, Paul M, Taksler G, et al. Heart failure-associated hospitalizations in the United States. J Am Coll Cardiol 2013;61(12):1259–67.
3. Heidenreich PA, Albert NM, Allen LA, et al. Forecasting the impact of heart failure in the United States: a policy statement from the American Heart Association. Circ Heart Fail 2013;6(3):606–19.
4. Javaheri S, Parker TJ, Liming JD, et al. Sleep apnea in 81 ambulatory male patients with stable heart failure. Types and their prevalences, consequences, and presentations. Circulation 1998; 97(21):2154–9.
5. Paulino A, Damy T, Margarit L, et al. Prevalence of sleep-disordered breathing in a 316-patient French

cohort of stable congestive heart failure. Arch Cardiovasc Dis 2009;102(3):169–75.

6. Oldenburg O, Lamp B, Faber L, et al. Sleep-disordered breathing in patients with symptomatic heart failure: a contemporary study of prevalence in and characteristics of 700 patients. Eur J Heart Fail 2007;9(3):251–7.

7. Lanfranchi PA, Somers VK, Braghiroli A, et al. Central sleep apnea in left ventricular dysfunction: prevalence and implications for arrhythmic risk. Circulation 2003;107(5):727–32.

8. Javaheri S, Blackwell T, Ancoli-Israel S, et al. Sleep-disordered breathing and incident heart failure in older men. Am J Respir Crit Care Med 2016; 193(5):561–8.

9. Gottlieb DJ, Yenokyan G, Newman AB, et al. Prospective study of obstructive sleep apnea and incident coronary heart disease and heart failure: the sleep heart health study. Circulation 2010;122(4):352–60.

10. Roca GQ, Redline S, Claggett B, et al. Sex-specific association of sleep apnea severity with Subclinical myocardial injury, ventricular hypertrophy, and heart failure risk in a community-Dwelling cohort: the Atherosclerosis risk in Communities-sleep heart health study. Circulation 2015; 132(14):1329–37.

11. Chan J, Sanderson J, Chan W, et al. Prevalence of sleep-disordered breathing in diastolic heart failure. Chest 1997;111(6):1488–93.

12. Javaheri S, Barbe F, Campos-Rodriguez F, et al. Sleep apnea: types, mechanisms, and clinical cardiovascular consequences. J Am Coll Cardiol 2017;69(7):841–58.

13. Khayat R, Jarjoura D, Porter K, et al. Sleep disordered breathing and post-discharge mortality in patients with acute heart failure. Eur Heart J 2015;36(23):1463–9.

14. Tkacova R, Wang H, Bradley TD. Night-to-night alterations in sleep apnea type in patients with heart failure. J Sleep Res 2006;15(3):321–8.

15. Osman AM, Carter SG, Carberry JC, et al. Obstructive sleep apnea: current perspectives. Nat Sci Sleep 2018;10:21–34.

16. Morgan BJ, Denahan T, Ebert TJ. Neurocirculatory consequences of negative intrathoracic pressure vs. asphyxia during voluntary apnea. J Appl Phys (1985) 1993;74(6):2969–75.

17. Katragadda S, Xie A, Puleo D, et al. Neural mechanism of the pressor response to obstructive and nonobstructive apnea. J Appl Physiol 1997;83(6): 2048–54.

18. Lesske J, Fletcher EC, Bao G, et al. Hypertension caused by chronic intermittent hypoxia–influence of chemoreceptors and sympathetic nervous system. J Hypertens 1997;15(12 Pt 2):1593–603.

19. Fletcher EC. Invited review: physiological consequences of intermittent hypoxia: systemic blood pressure. J Appl Physiol (1985) 2001;90(4): 1600–5.

20. Peppard PE, Young T, Palta M, et al. Prospective study of the association between sleep-disordered breathing and hypertension. N Engl J Med 2000;342(19):1378–84.

21. Leung RS, Bradley TD. Sleep apnea and cardiovascular disease. Am J Respir Crit Care Med 2001;164(12):2147–65.

22. Hung J, Whitford EG, Parsons RW, et al. Association of sleep apnoea with myocardial infarction in men. Lancet 1990;336(8710):261–4.

23. Franklin KA, Nilsson JB, Sahlin C, et al. Sleep apnoea and nocturnal angina. Lancet 1995; 345(8957):1085–7.

24. Peker Y, Hedner J, Kraiczi H, et al. Respiratory disturbance index: an independent predictor of mortality in coronary artery disease. Am J Respir Crit Care Med 2000;162(1):81–6.

25. Gami AS, Pressman G, Caples SM, et al. Association of atrial fibrillation and obstructive sleep apnea. Circulation 2004;110(4):364–7.

26. Bradley TD, Hall MJ, Ando S, et al. Hemodynamic effects of simulated obstructive apneas in humans with and without heart failure. Chest 2001;119(6): 1827–35.

27. Brinker JA, Weiss JL, Lappé DL, et al. Leftward septal displacement during right ventricular loading in man. Circulation 1980;61(3):626–33.

28. Arzt M, Young T, Finn L, et al. Sleepiness and sleep in patients with both systolic heart failure and obstructive sleep apnea. Arch Intern Med 2006; 166(16):1716–22.

29. Friedman O, Bradley TD, Chan CT, et al. Relationship between overnight rostral fluid shift and obstructive sleep apnea in drug-resistant hypertension. Hypertension 2010;56(6):1077–82.

30. Redolfi S, Yumino D, Ruttanaumpawan P, et al. Relationship between overnight rostral fluid shift and Obstructive Sleep Apnea in nonobese men. Am J Respir Crit Care Med 2009;179(3):241–6.

31. Naughton M, Benard D, Tam A, et al. Role of hyperventilation in the pathogenesis of central sleep apneas in patients with congestive heart failure. Am Rev Respir Dis 1993;148(2):330–8.

32. Xie A, Skatrud JB, Khayat R, et al. Cerebrovascular response to carbon dioxide in patients with congestive heart failure. Am J Respir Crit Care Med 2005;172(3):371–8.

33. Alex CG, Onal E, Lopata M. Upper airway occlusion during sleep in patients with Cheyne-Stokes respiration. Am Rev Respir Dis 1986;133(1):42–5.

34. Badr MS, Toiber F, Skatrud JB, et al. Pharyngeal narrowing/occlusion during central sleep apnea. J Appl Physiol (1985) 1995;78(5):1806–15.

35. Hall MJ, Xie A, Rutherford R, et al. Cycle length of periodic breathing in patients with and without

heart failure. Am J Respir Crit Care Med 1996; 154(2 Pt 1):376–81.

36. Somers VK, Mark AL, Zavala DC, et al. Contrasting effects of hypoxia and hypercapnia on ventilation and sympathetic activity in humans. J Appl Physiol (1985) 1989;67(5):2101–6.

37. Kaye DM, Lefkovits J, Jennings GL, et al. Adverse consequences of high sympathetic nervous activity in the failing human heart. J Am Coll Cardiol 1995; 26(5):1257–63.

38. Leung RS, Diep TM, Bowman ME, et al. Provocation of ventricular ectopy by cheyne-Stokes respiration in patients with heart failure. Sleep 2004; 27(7):1337–43.

39. Sin DD, Logan AG, Fitzgerald FS, et al. Effects of continuous positive airway pressure on cardiovascular outcomes in heart failure patients with and without Cheyne-Stokes respiration. Circulation 2000;102(1):61–6.

40. Lanfranchi PA, Braghiroli A, Bosimini E, et al. Prognostic value of nocturnal Cheyne-Stokes respiration in chronic heart failure. Circulation 1999; 99(11):1435–40.

41. Khayat R, Abraham W, Patt B, et al. Central sleep apnea is a predictor of cardiac readmission in hospitalized patients with systolic heart failure. J Card Fail 2012;18(7):534–40.

42. Mehra R, Wang L, Andrews N, et al. Dissociation of objective and subjective daytime sleepiness and biomarkers of systemic inflammation in sleep-disordered breathing and systolic heart failure. J Clin Sleep Med 2017;13(12):1411–22.

43. Sin DD, Fitzgerald F, Parker JD, et al. Risk factors for central and obstructive sleep apnea in 450 men and women with congestive heart failure. Am J Respir Crit Care Med 1999;160(4):1101–6.

44. MacDonald M, Fang J, Pittman SD, et al. The current prevalence of sleep disordered breathing in congestive heart failure patients treated with beta-blockers. J Clin Sleep Med 2008;4(1):38–42.

45. Tkacova R, Niroumand M, Lorenzi-Filho G, et al. Overnight shift from obstructive to central apneas in patients with heart failure: role of PCO2 and circulatory delay. Circulation 2001;103(2):238–43.

46. Kapur VK, Auckley DH, Chowdhuri S, et al. Clinical practice guideline for diagnostic testing for adult obstructive sleep apnea: an American Academy of sleep medicine clinical practice guideline. J Clin Sleep Med 2017;13(03):479–504.

47. Li S, Xu L, Dong X, et al. Home sleep apnea testing of adults with chronic heart failure. J Clin Sleep Med 2021;7(7):1453–63.

48. Patil SP, Ayappa IA, Caples SM, et al. Treatment of adult obstructive sleep apnea with positive airway pressure: an American Academy of sleep medicine clinical practice guideline. J Clin Sleep Med 2019; 15(2):335–43.

49. Chadda K, Annane D, Hart N, et al. Cardiac and respiratory effects of continuous positive airway pressure and noninvasive ventilation in acute cardiac pulmonary edema. Crit Care Med 2002; 30(11):2457–61.

50. Yoshinaga K, Burwash IG, Leech JA, et al. The effects of continuous positive airway pressure on myocardial energetics in patients with heart failure and obstructive sleep apnea. J Am Coll Cardiol 2007;49(4):450–8.

51. Naughton MT, Rahman MA, Hara K, et al. Effect of continuous positive airway pressure on intrathoracic and left ventricular transmural pressures in patients with congestive heart failure. Circulation 1995;91(6):1725–31.

52. Kasai T, Narui K, Dohi T, et al. Prognosis of patients with heart failure and obstructive sleep apnea treated with continuous positive airway pressure. Chest 2008;133(3):690–6.

53. Khayat RN, Abraham WT, Patt B, et al. In-hospital treatment of obstructive sleep apnea during decompensation of heart failure. Chest 2009; 136(4):991–7.

54. Spaak J, Egri ZJ, Kubo T, et al. Muscle sympathetic nerve activity during wakefulness in heart failure patients with and without sleep apnea. Hypertension 2005;46(6):1327–32.

55. Kaye DM, Mansfield D, Aggarwal A, et al. Acute effects of continuous positive airway pressure on cardiac sympathetic tone in congestive heart failure. Circulation 2001;103(19):2336–8.

56. Khoo MC, Belozeroff V, Berry RB, et al. Cardiac autonomic control in obstructive sleep apnea: effects of long-term CPAP therapy. Am J Respir Crit Care Med 2001;164(5):807–12.

57. Tkacova R, Rankin F, Fitzgerald FS, et al. Effects of continuous positive airway pressure on obstructive sleep apnea and left ventricular afterload in patients with heart failure. Circulation 1998;98(21):2269–75.

58. Sajkov D, Wang T, Saunders NA, et al. Continuous positive airway pressure treatment improves pulmonary hemodynamics in patients with obstructive sleep apnea. Am J Respir Crit Care Med 2002; 165(2):152–8.

59. Alchanatis M, Tourkohoriti G, Kakouros S, et al. Daytime pulmonary hypertension in patients with obstructive sleep apnea: the effect of continuous positive airway pressure on pulmonary hemodynamics. Respiration 2001;68(6):566–72.

60. Randerath W, Herkenrath S. Device therapy for sleep-disordered breathing in patients with cardiovascular diseases and heart failure. Sleep Med Clin 2017;12(2):243–54.

61. McEvoy RD, Antic NA, Heeley E, et al. CPAP for prevention of cardiovascular events in obstructive sleep apnea. N Engl J Med 2016;375(10): 919–31.

62. Martinez-Garcia MA, Campos-Rodriguez F, Javaheri S, et al. Pro: continuous positive airway pressure and cardiovascular prevention. Eur Respir J 2018;51(5):1702400.

63. Younes M. Apnea following mechanical ventilation may not Be caused by neuromechanical influences. Am J Respir Crit Care Med 2001;163(6): 1298–300.

64. Javaheri S, Brown LK, Abraham WT, et al. Apneas of heart failure and phenotype-guided treatments: Part One: OSA. Chest 2020;157(2):394–402.

65. Gottlieb DJ, Punjabi NM, Mehra R, et al. CPAP versus oxygen in obstructive sleep apnea. N Engl J Med 2014;370(24):2276–85.

66. Wellman A, Malhotra A, Jordan AS, et al. Effect of oxygen in obstructive sleep apnea: role of loop gain. Respir Physiol Neurobiol 2008;162(2):144–51.

67. Tojima H, Kunitomo F, Kimura H, et al. Effects of acetazolamide in patients with the sleep apnoea syndrome. Thorax 1988;43(2):113–9.

68. Edwards BA, Sands SA, Eckert DJ, et al. Acetazolamide improves loop gain but not the other physiological traits causing obstructive sleep apnoea. J Physiol 2012;590(5):1199–211.

69. Eckert DJ, Malhotra A, Wellman A, et al. Trazodone increases the respiratory arousal threshold in patients with obstructive sleep apnea and a low arousal threshold. Sleep 2014;37(4):811–9.

70. Rosenberg R, Roach JM, Scharf M, et al. A pilot study evaluating acute use of eszopiclone in patients with mild to moderate obstructive sleep apnea syndrome. Sleep Med 2007;8(5):464–70.

71. Eskafi M. Sleep apnoea in patients with stable congestive heart failure an intervention study with a mandibular advancement device. Swed Dent J Suppl 2004;(168):1–56.

72. Eskafi M, Cline C, Nilner M, et al. Treatment of sleep apnea in congestive heart failure with a dental device: the effect on brain natriuretic peptide and quality of life. Sleep Breath 2006;10(2): 90–7.

73. Servantes DM, Javaheri S, Kravchychyn ACP, et al. Effects of exercise training and CPAP in patients with heart failure and OSA: a Preliminary study. Chest 2018;154(4):808–17.

74. Ueno LM, Drager LF, Rodrigues ACT, et al. Effects of exercise training in patients with chronic heart failure and sleep apnea. Sleep 2009;32(5):637–47.

75. Li YL, Ding Y, Agnew C, et al. Exercise training improves peripheral chemoreflex function in heart failure rabbits. J Appl Physiol (1985) 2008;105(3): 782–90.

76. Tomita T, Takaki H, Hara Y, et al. Attenuation of hypercapnic carbon dioxide chemosensitivity after postinfarction exercise training: possible contribution to the improvement in exercise hyperventilation. Heart 2003;89(4):404–10.

77. Guimaraes KC, Drager LF, Genta PR, et al. Effects of oropharyngeal exercises on patients with moderate obstructive sleep apnea syndrome. Am J Respir Crit Care Med 2009;179(10):962–6.

78. Solin P, Bergin P, Richardson M, et al. Influence of pulmonary capillary wedge pressure on central apnea in heart failure. Circulation 1999;99(12):1574–9.

79. Javaheri S, Abraham WT, Brown C, et al. Prevalence of obstructive sleep apnoea and periodic limb movement in 45 subjects with heart transplantation. Eur Heart J 2004;25(3):260–6.

80. van de Borne P, Oren R, Abouassaly C, et al. Effect of Cheyne-Stokes respiration on muscle sympathetic nerve activity in severe congestive heart failure secondary to ischemic or idiopathic dilated cardiomyopathy. Am J Cardiol 1998; 81(4):432–6.

81. Toyama T, Seki R, Kasama S, et al. Effectiveness of nocturnal home oxygen therapy to improve exercise capacity, cardiac function and cardiac sympathetic nerve activity in patients with chronic heart failure and central sleep apnea. Circ J 2009; 73(2):299–304.

82. Naughton MT, Benard DC, Liu PP, et al. Effects of nasal CPAP on sympathetic activity in patients with heart failure and central sleep apnea. Am J Respir Crit Care Med 1995;152(2):473–9.

83. Ponikowski P, Chua TP, Anker SD, et al. Peripheral chemoreceptor hypersensitivity: an ominous sign in patients with chronic heart failure. Circulation 2001;104(5):544–9.

84. Javaheri S. Pembrey's dream: the time has come for a long-term trial of nocturnal supplemental nasal oxygen to treat central sleep apnea in congestive heart failure. Chest 2003;123(2):322–5.

85. Javaheri S, Ahmed M, Parker TJ, et al. Effects of nasal O2 on sleep-related disordered breathing in ambulatory patients with stable heart failure. Sleep 1999;22(8):1101–6.

86. Oldenburg O, Wellmann B, Buchholz A, et al. Nocturnal hypoxaemia is associated with increased mortality in stable heart failure patients. Eur Heart J 2016;37(21):1695–703.

87. Staniforth AD, Kinnear WJ, Starling R, et al. Effect of oxygen on sleep quality, cognitive function and sympathetic activity in patients with chronic heart failure and Cheyne-Stokes respiration. Eur Heart J 1998;19(6):922–8.

88. Andreas S, Bingeli C, Mohacsi P, et al. Nasal oxygen and muscle sympathetic nerve activity in heart failure. Chest 2003;123(2):366–71.

89. Sasayama S, Izumi T, Selno Y, et al. Effects of nocturnal oxygen therapy on outcome measures in patients with chronic heart failure and cheyne-Stokes respiration. Circ J 2006;70(1):1–7.

90. Sasayama S, Izumi T, Matsuzaki M, et al. Improvement of quality of life with nocturnal oxygen therapy

in heart failure patients with central sleep apnea. Circ J 2009;73(7):1255–62.

91. Clark AL, Johnson M, Fairhurst C, et al. Does home oxygen therapy (HOT) in addition to standard care reduce disease severity and improve symptoms in people with chronic heart failure? A randomised trial of home oxygen therapy for patients with chronic heart failure. Health Technol Assess 2015; 19(75):1–120.

92. Daly WJ, Bondurant S. Effects of oxygen breathing on the heart rate, blood pressure, and cardiac index of normal men–resting, with reactive hyperemia, and after atropine. J Clin Invest 1962;41(1): 126–32.

93. Mak S, Azevedo ER, Liu PP, et al. Effect of hyperoxia on left ventricular function and filling pressures in patients with and without congestive heart failure. Chest 2001;120(2):467–73.

94. Haque WA, Boehmer J, Clemson BS, et al. Hemodynamic effects of supplemental oxygen administration in congestive heart failure. J Am Coll Cardiol 1996;27(2):353–7.

95. Nakayama H, Smith CA, Rodman JR, et al. Effect of ventilatory drive on carbon dioxide sensitivity below eupnea during sleep. Am J Respir Crit Care Med 2002;165(9):1251–60.

96. Lyons OD, Bradley TD. Heart failure and sleep apnea. Can J Cardiol 2015;31(7):898–908.

97. Dempsey JA. Crossing the apnoeic threshold: causes and consequences. Exp Physiol 2005; 90(1):13–24.

98. Javaheri S, Parker TJ, Wexler L, et al. Effect of theophylline on sleep-disordered breathing in heart failure. N Engl J Med 1996;335(8):562–7.

99. Del Rio R, Marcus NJ, Schultz HD. Carotid chemoreceptor ablation improves survival in heart failure: rescuing autonomic control of cardiorespiratory function. J Am Coll Cardiol 2013;62(25):2422–30.

100. Marcus NJ, Del Rio R, Schultz HD. Central role of carotid body chemoreceptors in disordered breathing and cardiorenal dysfunction in chronic heart failure. Front Physiol 2014;5:438.

101. Niewinski P, Janczak D, Rucinski A, et al. Carotid body removal for treatment of chronic systolic heart failure. Int J Cardiol 2013;168(3):2506–9.

102. Niewinski P, Janczak D, Rucinski A, et al. Carotid body resection for sympathetic modulation in systolic heart failure: results from first-in-man study. Eur J Heart Fail 2017;19(3):391–400.

103. Biberdorf DJ, Steens R, Millar TW, et al. Benzodiazepines in congestive heart failure: effects of temazepam on arousability and Cheyne-Stokes respiration. Sleep 1993;16(6):529–38.

104. Dowdell WT, Javaheri S, McGinnis W. Cheyne-Stokes respiration presenting as sleep apnea syndrome. Clinical and polysomnographic features. Am Rev Respir Dis 1990;141(4 Pt 1):871–9.

105. Cartwright RD, Samelson CF. The effects of a nonsurgical treatment for obstructive sleep apnea. The tongue-retaining device. JAMA 1982;248(6): 705–9.

106. Kuzniar TJ, Kovacevic-Ristanovic R, Freedom T. Complex sleep apnea unmasked by the use of a mandibular advancement device. Sleep Breath 2011;15(2):249–52.

107. Bradley TD, Logan AG, Kimoff RJ, et al. Continuous positive airway pressure for central sleep apnea and heart failure. N Engl J Med 2005;353(19): 2025–33.

108. Arzt M, Floras JS, Logan AG, et al. Suppression of central sleep apnea by continuous positive airway pressure and transplant-free survival in heart failure: a post hoc analysis of the Canadian Continuous Positive Airway Pressure for Patients with Central Sleep Apnea and Heart Failure Trial (CANPAP). Circulation 2007;115(25):3173–80.

109. Sands SA, Edwards BA, Kee K, et al. Loop gain as a means to predict a positive airway pressure suppression of Cheyne-Stokes respiration in patients with heart failure. Am J Respir Crit Care Med 2011;184(9):1067–75.

110. Javaheri S, Brown LK, Randerath WJ. Positive airway pressure therapy with adaptive servoventilation: part 1: operational algorithms. Chest 2014; 146(2):514–23.

111. Aurora RN, Chowdhuri S, Ramar K, et al. The treatment of central sleep apnea syndromes in adults: practice parameters with an evidence-based literature review and meta-analyses. Sleep 2012;35(1): 17–40.

112. Cowie MR, Woehrle H, Wegscheider K, et al. Adaptive servo-ventilation for central sleep apnea in systolic heart failure. N Engl J Med 2015;373(12): 1095–105.

113. Aurora RN, Bista SR, Casey KR, et al. Updated adaptive servo-ventilation recommendations for the 2012 AASM guideline: "the treatment of central sleep apnea syndromes in adults: practice parameters with an evidence-based literature review and meta-analyses. J Clin Sleep Med 2016;12(5): 757–61.

114. Cowie MR, Woehrle H, Wegscheider K, et al. Adaptive servo-ventilation for central sleep apnoea in systolic heart failure: results of the major substudy of SERVE-HF. Eur J Heart Fail 2018; 20(3):536–44.

115. Floras JS, Logan AG, Bradley TD. Adaptive servo ventilation for central sleep apnea: more data, please. Can J Cardiol 2016;32(3):396. e393.

116. Adaptive servo-ventilation for central sleep apnea in heart failure. N Engl J Med 2016;374(7):687–91.

117. Bradley TD, Floras JS. Adaptive servo-ventilation and the treatment of central sleep apnea in heart failure. Let's not throw the baby out with the

bathwater. Am J Respir Crit Care Med 2015;193(4): 357–9.

118. Douglas Bradley T, Floras JS, The A-HFI. The SERVE-HF trial. Can Respir J : J Can Thorac Soc 2015;22(6):313.

119. Woehrle H, Cowie MR, Eulenburg C, et al. Adaptive servo ventilation for central sleep apnoea in heart failure: SERVE-HF on-treatment analysis. Eur Respir J 2017;50(2):1601692.

120. Lyons OD, Floras JS, Logan AG, et al. Design of the effect of adaptive servo-ventilation on survival and cardiovascular hospital admissions in patients with heart failure and sleep apnoea: the ADVENT-HF trial. Eur J Heart Fail 2017;19(4):579–87.

121. Hetland A, Lerum TV, Haugaa KH, et al. Patients with Cheyne-Stokes respiration and heart failure: patient tolerance after three-month discontinuation of treatment with adaptive servo-ventilation. Heart Vessels 2017;32(8):909–15.

122. Olseng Margareth W, Olsen Brita F, Hetland A, et al. Quality of life improves in patients with chronic heart failure and Cheyne-Stokes respiration treated with adaptive servo-ventilation in a nurse-led heart failure clinic. J Clin Nurs 2017;26(9–10): 1226–33.

123. Yoshida M, Ando S-i, Kodama K, et al. Adaptive servo-ventilation therapy reduces hospitalization rate in patients with severe heart failure. Int J Cardiol 2017;238:173–6.

124. Hiasa G, Okayama H, Hosokawa S, et al. Beneficial effects of adaptive servo-ventilation therapy on readmission and medical costs in patients with chronic heart failure. Heart and vessels 2018; 33(8):859–65.

125. Chen ML, Tablizo MA, Kun S, et al. Diaphragm pacers as a treatment for congenital central hypoventilation syndrome. Expert Rev Med Devices 2005;2(5):577–85.

126. DiMarco AF. Phrenic nerve stimulation in patients with spinal cord injury. Respir Physiol Neurobiol 2009;169(2):200–9.

127. Glenn WW, Brouillette RT, Dentz B, et al. Fundamental considerations in pacing of the diaphragm for chronic ventilatory insufficiency: a multi-center study. Pacing Clin Electrophysiol 1988;11(11 Pt 2):2121–7.

128. Ponikowski P, Javaheri S, Michalkiewicz D, et al. Transvenous phrenic nerve stimulation for the treatment of central sleep apnoea in heart failure. Eur Heart J 2012;33(7):889–94.

129. Costanzo MR, Augostini R, Goldberg LR, et al. Design of the remede system pivotal trial: a prospective, randomized study in the Use of respiratory rhythm management to treat central sleep apnea. J Card Fail 2015;21(11):892–902.

130. Jagielski D, Ponikowski P, Augostini R, et al. Transvenous stimulation of the phrenic nerve for the treatment of central sleep apnoea: 12 months' experience with the remede((R)) System. Eur J Heart Fail 2016;18(11):1386–93.

131. Zhang X, Ding N, Ni B, et al. Safety and feasibility of chronic transvenous phrenic nerve stimulation for treatment of central sleep apnea in heart failure patients. Clin Respir J 2017;11(2):176–84.

Sleep-Related Breathing Complaints in Chronic Obstructive Pulmonary Disease

Albert L. Rafanan, MD, FCCP, FASSM, FPSSM, FPCP, FPCCP, DABSM[a,b,c,*],
Rylene A. Baquilod, MD, FPCP, FPCCP, FPSSM[c]

KEYWORDS

- Sleep • COPD • Sleep-related breathing disorders • Overlap syndrome • Nocturnal desaturation
- Long-term nocturnal noninvasive ventilation

KEY POINTS

- Normal physiologic changes in respiration can predispose to SRBDs in COPD.
- The diagnosis of OS requires a high index of suspicion and routine assessment is needed as this is associated with worse prognosis; and treatment with positive airway pressure reduces mortality.
- Oxygen supplementation for isolated nocturnal oxygen desaturation does not decrease mortality or progression of disease.
- Long-term nocturnal noninvasive ventilation is recommended for patients with chronic stable hypercapnic.

BACKGROUND

There is a global increase of chronic obstructive pulmonary disease (COPD) with a worldwide estimated prevalence of 13.1%.[1] COPD is currently one of the top 3 causes of death worldwide.[2] COPD is a chronic inflammatory lung disease characterized by persistent airflow limitation due to airway and/or alveolar abnormalities caused by significant exposure to noxious particles or gases.[3] Spirometry is essential for a diagnosis of COPD with a postbronchodilator FEV1/FVC ratio less than 0.7.[3]

Patients with COPD are often affected by respiratory symptoms, such as chronic and progressive dyspnea, cough, or sputum production. Comorbidities such as cardiovascular disease, sarcopenia, osteoporosis, depression, and lung cancer are frequently seen. These comorbidities contribute to a higher risk of adverse outcomes of mortality and hospitalizations in COPD.[4] Sleep disorders are also major comorbidity, and these often remain unrecognized and unresolved as the assessment of the patient's sleep is not routinely part of our follow-up of patients with COPD.[5]

Sleep is associated with physiologic changes that may be detrimental to COPD.[6] Sleep complaints are common in COPD with some reports citing as much as 40%.[7–10] Sleep disturbance in COPD can be caused by disease-specific symptoms, medications, and the presence of sleep disorders, and other medical and psychological conditions.[11,12] Sleep disorders may worsen the quality of life and increase the odds of adverse health outcomes, including mortality.[9,13–15]

Sleep has several critical effects on the respiratory system and gas exchange which may worsen the breathing in COPD.[8,16] The symptoms of sleep-related breathing disorders (SRBDs) in patients with COPD can manifest as gas exchange abnormalities, insomnia, snoring, fatigue, daytime

[a] Center for Sleep Disorders, Critical Care Committee, Chong Hua Hospital, Cebu City, Philippines; [b] Cebu Doctors University College of Medicine, Cebu City, Philippines; [c] Pulmonary and Pulmonary Critical Care, Chong Hua Hospital, Cebu City, Philippines
* Corresponding author. Chong Hua Hospital Medical Arts Building, Room 110, J Llorente St., Cebu City, Philippines.
E-mail address: rafananalbert@gmail.com

Sleep Med Clin 17 (2022) 99–109
https://doi.org/10.1016/j.jsmc.2021.10.008
1556-407X/22/© 2021 Elsevier Inc. All rights reserved.

Abbreviations	
OS	Overlap Syndrome
SRDBs	Sleep Related Breathing Disorders
COPD	Chronic Obstructive Pulmonary Disease
LTOT	Long-Term Oxygen Treatment
NOT	Nocturnal Oxygen Therapy

sleepiness, and increased arousals.[17–19] SRBDs are frequently seen with COPD and need to be addressed as it can lead to higher economic cost and increased rates of morbidity and mortality.[20–23]

PHYSIOLOGICAL CHANGES IN VENTILATION DURING SLEEP

During the different stages of sleep, there is marked respiratory variability as a result of a change in the central neural control drive and to a decreased tone of the upper airway muscles and the respiratory muscles[24,25] (**Fig. 1**). In normal individuals, this collection of adverse events is of insignificant consequence.

Effect of Sleep on the Central Control of Breathing

In the awake state, breathing is regulated by 3 major feedbacks: (1) voluntary control and behavioral information from higher cortical centers that allows breathing to be regulated in activities such as singing, speaking, and eating; (2) chemical factors (eg, acidosis, carbon dioxide, and oxygen levels); and (3) mechanical signals from the lung and chest wall. During sleep, most of the inputs capable of modifying breathing are markedly downregulated or absent. The higher cortical centers cease to modify breathing with sleep onset. The chemical control of breathing is the dominant input to ventilatory control during sleep and aims to regulate the respiratory system to normalize blood gases, particularly the partial pressure of arterial CO2 ($Paco_2$).[26]

During sleep, there is a blunted ventilatory response to both hypoxemia and hypercapnia and are their lowest during rapid eye movement (REM) sleep.[24] The hypercapnic ventilatory response is decreased from wakefulness to non-rapid eye movement (NREM) sleep by about 50%.[27,28] During REM sleep, the hypercapnic ventilatory response is only 28% when compared with the awake state.[27] Individuals are able to tolerate a higher level of $Paco_2$ during sleep than in wakefulness, and the $Paco_2$ may increase by 3 mm Hg during sleep.[27] Similarly, the ventilatory response to hypoxia falls during sleep. The hypoxic ventilatory response is lower during NREM sleep in men, but not in women.[27,29,30] During REM sleep, there is a decreased response to hypoxia in both sexes by about 0.4/L/min/percentage SaO_2.[27,30]

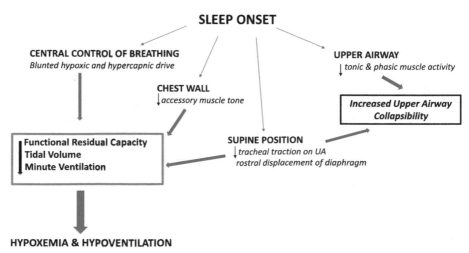

Fig. 1. Physiologic effects of sleep on respiratory ventilation.

Impact of Sleep on the Upper Airway

To effect normal respiration, the airway should remain patent throughout the respiratory cycle. The mechanical properties of the upper airway are markedly affected by sleep. Loss of the wakefulness stimulus induces a significant reduction in both the tonic and phasic upper airway muscle activity.[31,32] This results in an increased upper airway resistance from a decreased upper airway size and compliance.[32] In addition, supine position during sleep causes rostral displacement of the diaphragm by abdominal contents reducing the functional residual capacity, and also decreasing caudal traction on the upper airway.[33] Sleep impairs upper airway muscle control and affects chest wall mechanics predisposing to a more collapsible upper airway leading to obstructive respiratory events during sleep.

Effect of Sleep on the Chest Wall

Generalized muscle hypotonia occurs throughout sleep being most profound during REM sleep when there is almost a complete loss of tone of the intercostal muscles. There is relative preservation of diaphragmatic tone and there is reliance on this muscle for the maintenance of ventilation especially during REM sleep.[34] This inspiratory muscle hypotonia may cause a decrease in minute ventilation in diseases, in which accessory respiratory muscles contribute substantially to ventilation.[25]

PATHOPHYSIOLOGY OF SLEEP-RELATED BREATHING DISORDERS IN CHRONIC OBSTRUCTIVE PULMONARY DISEASE

Physiologic changes in respiration during sleep usually do not lead to any significant detriment in healthy individuals; but in patients with COPD, there may be profound respiratory derangements causing significant hypoxemia and hypercarbia.[35] Nocturnal oxygen desaturation occurs in 27% to 70% of patients even in the absence of upper airway obstruction.[19,36,37] Nocturnal desaturation in patients with COPD is most significantly linked with baseline awake hypoxemia.[19] When the resting oxygen saturation levels are on the steep portion of the oxyhemoglobin dissociation curve, there will be a larger decline in the oxygen saturation during sleep.[38] Sleep causes greater derangement in patients with COPD with poorer lung function.

Generalized muscle hypotonia occurs throughout sleep, and especially during REM sleep, wherein the diaphragm may be the sole muscle for maintenance of ventilation.[34]

Hypoventilation and oxygen desaturation may occur in patients with severe COPD who are dependent on their accessory muscles to maintain ventilation.[39,40] Furthermore, hypoventilation occurs due to a decreased ventilatory response to hypoxia and hypercarbia in sleep.[27,28,35] Ventilation may be 40% lower in REM than in the awake state.[41]

Patients with COPD have irreversible lung disease with variable air trapping and dynamic hyperinflation.[42] During wakefulness, patients with COPD adopt specific mechanisms to offset dynamic hyperinflation and preserve alveolar ventilation, including extending expiratory time and pursed-lip breathing.[43,44] In sleep, there can be a marked increase in the $Paco_2$ in COPD due to a reduction in ventilation and concurrent increase in dead space ventilation.[45]

Lung hyperinflation in patients with COPD and the supine position reduces the efficiency of the diaphragm, leading to further reduction of the tidal volume.[40] The decrease in the end-expiratory volume will lead to an increase in physiologic dead space in COPD leading to further deterioration of pulmonary gas exchange and accentuating the sleep-related hypoventilation.[39,45] V/Q mismatch also increases due to increased airway resistance and closing of the small airways in the dependent lung.[41,46] The collective effect of these mechanisms is a persistent and dramatic nocturnal desaturation especially during REM sleep.[47,48]

SPECIFIC SLEEP-RELATED BREATHING DISORDERS IN CHRONIC OBSTRUCTIVE PULMONARY DISEASE AND THEIR PROGNOSTIC IMPLICATIONS
Overlap Syndrome

Prevalence
Obstructive sleep apnea (OSA) is a disorder characterized by obstructive apneas, and hypopneas caused by repetitive collapse of the upper airway during sleep.[49] It is the most common SRBDs with a prevalence of at least 10% in the general population.[50,51] The term "overlap syndrome" (OS) has been used to refer to the coexistence of both COPD and OSA in the same patient.[52,53] The prevalence rate of OS ranges from 1% to 4% of the general population[52,54–57] In patients with OSA, the presence of OS is 7.6% to 55.7%.[56,58–60] Among patients with COPD, the prevalence of OS ranges from 2.9% to 65.9%.[56,61,62] The wide range of prevalence may reflect the methodological diversity in the definitions and diagnostic techniques used to diagnose OSA and COPD.[56]

Pathophysiology of overlap syndrome

As both COPD and OSA are remarkably common in the adult population, they can occur quite frequently in the same individual and both can coexist without necessarily having an epidemiologic or causal relationship.[54,63] However, evidence does show that there is a reciprocal interaction, whereby COPD and OSA impacts the severity of its comorbidities[64–66]

There are COPD-related factors that may lead to the development of OS (Fig. 2). Advanced age is associated with the prevalence of OS and it is seen in up to 64% of COPD with an age more than 70.[67] Compared with OSA by itself, patients with OS were also found to have an advanced age.[58,60,68] Obesity is a major factor with around 50% of patients with OSA are obese.[69,70] Patients with COPD with a higher body mass index (BMI) are at increased risk for OSA.[71]

OS is more common in the chronic bronchitis phenotype of COPD as these patients have a higher BMI, cor pulmonale with edema, and more likely to have hypoxemia and hypercarbia.[72] The predominantly emphysema phenotype is thought to be of lower risk for OSA, as these patients often have sarcopenia and have a lower BMI.[72] The increased lung volumes seen with emphysema are thought to be protective against OSA as it lowers the critical closing pressure of the upper airway during sleep.[73]

Cigarette smoking predisposes to OS by increasing upper airway resistance due to local inflammation and edema.[74] Current heavy smokers have a greater likelihood of snoring and SRBDs than never and former smokers.[75] An increased pack-year smoking history also increases the risk for OSA.[71] Former smoking was not associated with OS; thus, all should be encouraged to stop smoking.[75]

The severity of the disease also affects the development of OS. Patients with COPD requiring long-term oxygen therapy were found to have a higher incidence of OS.[62,67] Patients with cor pulmonale or has edema from heart failure have rostral fluid shift into the neck in the supine position; this may promote pharyngeal collapsibility and OSA.[76] Patients with COPD with repeated or chronic steroid use may develop myopathy and accumulation of fat in the parapharyngeal tissues, both of which can increase upper airway collapsibility.[74]

Prognostic implications

Both COPD and OSA are associated with airway and systemic inflammation which is implicated as an important mechanism in the development of cardiovascular complications.[74] Patients with OS have more episodes of oxygen desaturation and longer sleep time with hypoxemia and hypercarbia than OSA without COPD.[58] This added burden of repetitive hypoxemia seen in OSA with COPD may be an important mechanism of cardiovascular morbidity contributing to increases in systemic and pulmonary blood pressure and occurrence of arrhythmias.[77,78]

In a large cross-sectional study consisting of a population of more than 16,000 patients, Adler and colleagues found that patients with OS have a more severe course of SDB than OSA, as they have a higher apnea–hypopnea index (AHI), higher oxygen desaturation index (ODI), and a lower mean nocturnal oxygen saturation.[66] Patients with OS were also found to have an increased prevalence of coronary heart disease, heart failure,

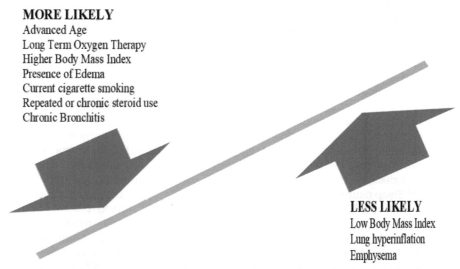

MORE LIKELY
Advanced Age
Long Term Oxygen Therapy
Higher Body Mass Index
Presence of Edema
Current cigarette smoking
Repeated or chronic steroid use
Chronic Bronchitis

LESS LIKELY
Low Body Mass Index
Lung hyperinflation
Emphysema

Fig. 2. Clinical factors that make it more likely and less likely for COPD to have concomitant obstructive sleep apnea.

and peripheral arteriopathy.[66] There is also an increased incidence of pulmonary hypertension. Others have also reported that pulmonary hypertension occurs in 50% to 82% of patients with OS compared with only 13% to 16% in patients with OSA.[58,79]

Overlap syndrome has also been reported as a major cause of ICU admissions.[80] Patients with OS have more severe respiratory symptoms with increased exacerbations and hospitalizations.[81,82] All-cause mortality is higher in patients with untreated OS than in those with COPD or OSA alone.[83,84] Patients with OS often die from cardiovascular complications.[83]

Diagnosis and treatment

The clinical symptoms of OS are sleepiness, increased arousals, snoring, and gas exchange abnormalities. They are also frequently seen in patients with COPD. Some patients with OS may also be minimally symptomatic.[66] Questionnaires for screening OSA have not been validated in COPD and do not accurately predict OS.[85] The usual risk factors such as male gender, neck circumference, and BMI are inconsistently associated with OSA in COPD.[85,86] The diagnosis of OS requires a high index of suspicion.

When OSA is suspected, overnight pulse oximetry monitoring is not a reliable screening tool.[87,88] Home sleep apnea test (HSAT) is also not recommended for the diagnosis of OSA in patients with significant cardiorespiratory disease or suspicion of sleep-related hypoventilation.[89] Only a minority (36%) of HSAT in COPD were of reasonable quality for interpretation.[90] When OS is suspected, a full-night, in-laboratory polysomnogram (PSG) should be obtained, unless the COPD is mild and the sleep quality is good.[35] PSG is the gold standard method for the diagnosis of OSA and other forms of SRBDs. Evaluation of COPD with a PSG is warranted when there is a clinical suspicion of sleep apnea or complications of hypoxemia that are not explained by the awake arterial oxygen levels, and pulmonary hypertension out of proportion to the severity of pulmonary function derangement.[91]

Treatment goals in OS are aimed at reducing obstructive respiratory events, improving gas exchange, and improving sleep quality. Oxygen supplementation alone is not recommended as it may increase the duration of obstructive respiratory events and worsen respiratory acidosis.[92,93] Continuous positive airway pressure (CPAP) therapy remains the mainstay of therapy for OSA in adults. Initiation of CPAP in patients with OS generally follows the same protocol used for routine treatment of OSA alone. In patients with OS, CPAP therapy has been shown to decrease

mortality.[62,83] Patients who are more compliant with their CPAP achieve greater benefit as usage time is independently associated with survival.[57] CPAP in OS has also been shown to decrease COPD exacerbations and hospitalization.[83,94] CPAP was also shown to significantly improve lung function and gas exchange parameters.[95,96] The improvement in lung function was particularly superior in the group of patients with OS who were hypercapnic.[95] Screening for OSA in patients with COPD is imperative as mortality can be improved with appropriate intervention.

Nocturnal Hypoxemia

Nocturnal desaturation is usually defined as a $SpO_2 \leq 88\%$ for more than one-third of the night.[97,98] Nocturnal desaturation in patients with COPD, not associated with obstructive apneas or hypopneas, may occur before severe daytime hypoxemia develops.[48,99–101] Currently, long-term oxygen treatment (LTOT) is only recommended for severe awake hypoxemia and not for moderate chronic resting room air hypoxemia or isolated nocturnal oxygen desaturation.[97,102,103]

In patients receiving LTOT for severe hypoxemia, the prescribed oxygen requirements during the awake state may be inadequate, as nocturnal oxygen saturation may fall to less than 90%.[104–106] It is recommended that the flow rate be increased by 1 L/min during sleep in patients with nonhypercapnic COPD.[102,107] Monitoring nocturnal pulse oximetry is best as it allows for more accurate flow rates during sleep.[104,105]

It is estimated that isolated nocturnal desaturation without severe awake hypoxemia occurs in less than 5% of all patients with COPD.[108] However, when the awake resting saturation is less than 95%, approximately half will have significant nocturnal desaturation.[108] Moreover, in a cross-sectional study of moderate to severe COPD with mild-to-moderate daytime hypoxemia, almost 40% had nocturnal desaturation without evidence of sleep apnea.[99]

Nocturnal oxygen therapy (NOT) is the administration of oxygen during sleep alone without additional oxygen therapy during the awake state. Treatment of isolated nocturnal desaturation is believed by some clinicians to be beneficial as some studies have shown that untreated oxygen desaturation during sleep can increase mortality, promote neuronal damage, and predispose to respiratory failure, cardiovascular disease, and pulmonary hypertension.[97,109–115]

Four randomized trials have been published to determine the benefit of NOT, and none was able to show evidence of improved survival or delay in the progression of the disease.[111,116–118] The largest of this trial is the International Nocturnal Oxygen (INOX) trial, which randomized 243 patients.[118] Unfortunately, the study was underpowered as enrollment had to be stopped because of recruitment and retention difficulties. An updated meta-analysis conducted by the authors of the INOX trial still did not provide evidence of benefit from the use of NOT with COPD and isolated nocturnal desaturation.[118] Current evidence does not support the use of NOT in COPD with isolated nocturnal desaturation as it does not decrease mortality or prevent progression of the disease. However, NOT may be beneficial in certain phenotypes of COPD. For instance, it was shown that NOT is beneficial in moderate to severe patients with COPD during high altitude travel as it significantly improves nocturnal breathing disturbances and other altitude-related adverse health effects.[119] More trials are needed to determine if NOT will be beneficial in other important endpoints aside from mortality. Will the use of NOT in COPD improve health-related quality of life, cognitive function, or exercise capacity? Will the use of NOT in COPD decrease or prevent cardiovascular morbidities, pulmonary hypertension, exacerbations, or hospitalizations?

Long-Term Nocturnal Noninvasive Ventilation

Sleep-related hypoventilation, defined as an increase in $Paco_2$ to greater than 55 mm Hg or rise in $Paco_2$ by $\geq$ 10 mm Hg from wake value to a level $\geq$ 50 mm Hg for at least 10 minutes during sleep, has a prevalence of about 6% to 10% and is often limited to REM sleep in patients with mild COPD. However, prevalence can be as high as 43% in hypercapnic patients with COPD.[13,120]

Noninvasive ventilation is an established therapy during acute exacerbations of COPD.[121] There has been a growing interest in the use of long-term nocturnal NIV in chronic stable hypercapnic COPD, as these patients are more prone to decline in health and have a higher mortality.[122,123] The use of nocturnal NIV may reduce lung hyperinflation, decrease respiratory muscle workload, and improve respiratory center's sensitivity to CO2.[124–126]

Both the American Thoracic Society and European Respiratory Society have released guidelines on the use of long-term nocturnal NIV for chronic hypercapnic COPD.[127,128] Thirteen randomized controlled trials were evaluated. Long-term nocturnal NIV decreased mortality by 14% (95% confidence interval (CI): 0.58–1.27), resulted

in 1.26 fewer hospitalizations (95% CI: 0.08–2.59), improved quality of life and dyspnea compared with standard of care.[127,128] Both guidelines suggest the use of nocturnal long-term NIV in addition to usual care for patients with chronic stable hypercapnic COPD.[127,128] It is also recommended that these patients should first undergo assessment for sleep apnea.[127,128] Initiation of NIV need not be conducted using PSG, but it is suggested that NIV setting be titrated to normalize or at least cause a significant reduction in $Paco_2$.[127,128]

SUMMARY

In COPD, SRBDs are quite common. Clinicians need to routinely evaluate patients with COPD for sleep complaints as treatment of SRBDs will contribute to a significant reduction of morbidity, exacerbation frequency, and mortality.

CLINICS CARE POINTS

- Sleep complaints are common in COPD, and failure to treat SRBDs will lead to increased cost and higher rates of morbidity and mortality.

- Normal physiologic respiratory changes during sleep may lead to profound respiratory derangements in patients with COPD.

- Treatment of overlap syndrome with CPAP decreases mortality, exacerbations, and hospitalizations.

- Oxygen therapy in patients with COPD with isolated nocturnal desaturation does not decrease mortality.

- Long-term nocturnal noninvasive ventilation in chronic stable hypercapnic COPD decreases mortality and hospitalizations.

DISCLOSURE

The authors have nothing to disclose.

REFERENCES

1. Blanco I, Diego I, Bueno P, et al. Geographic distribution of COPD prevalence in the world displayed by Geographic Information System maps. Eur Respir J 2019;54(1).
2. Halpin DMG, Celli BR, Criner GJ, et al. The GOLD Summit on chronic obstructive pulmonary disease in low- and middle-income countries. Int J Tuberc Lung Dis 2019;23(11):1131–41.

3. Global Initiative for Chronic Obstructive Lung Disease (GOLD). Global strategy for the diagnosis, management, and prevention of chronic obstructive pulmonary disease. 2021. Available at: www.goldcopd.org. Accessed May 25, 2021.

4. Mannino DM, Thorn D, Swensen A, et al. Prevalence and outcomes of diabetes, hypertension and cardiovascular disease in COPD. Eur Respir J 2008;32(4):962–9.

5. Lal C, Kumbhare S, Strange C. Prevalence of self-reported sleep problems amongst adults with obstructive airway disease in the NHANES cohort in the United States. Sleep Breath 2020;24(3):985–93.

6. Grandner MA. Sleep, health, and society. Sleep Med Clin 2020;15(2):319–40.

7. Budhiraja R, Parthasarathy S, Budhiraja P, et al. Insomnia in patients with COPD. Sleep 2012;35(3):369–75.

8. Rennard S, Decramer M, Calverley PM, et al. Impact of COPD in North America and Europe in 2000: subjects' perspective of Confronting COPD International survey. Eur Respir J 2002;20(4):799–805.

9. Lee SH, Lee H, Kim YS, et al. Factors associated with sleep disturbance in patients with chronic obstructive pulmonary disease. Clin Respir J 2020;14(11):1018–24.

10. Vaidya S, Gothi D, Patro M. Prevalence of sleep disorders in chronic obstructive pulmonary disease and utility of global sleep assessment questionnaire: an observational case-control study. Ann Thorac Med 2020;15(4):230–7.

11. Agusti A, Hedner J, Marin JM, et al. Night-time symptoms: a forgotten dimension of COPD. Eur Respir Rev 2011;20(121):183–94.

12. Collop N. Sleep and sleep disorders in chronic obstructive pulmonary disease. Respiration 2010;80(1):78–86.

13. Budhiraja R, Siddiqi TA, Quan SF. Sleep disorders in chronic obstructive pulmonary disease: etiology, impact, and management. J Clin Sleep Med 2015;11(3):259–70.

14. Ding B, Small M, Bergstrom G, et al. A cross-sectional survey of night-time symptoms and impact of sleep disturbance on symptoms and health status in patients with COPD. Int J Chron Obstruct Pulmon Dis 2017;12:589–99.

15. Omachi TA, Blanc PD, Claman DM, et al. Disturbed sleep among COPD patients is longitudinally associated with mortality and adverse COPD outcomes. Sleep Med 2012;13(5):476–83.

16. Newton K, Malik V, Lee-Chiong T. Sleep and breathing. Clin Chest Med 2014;35(3):451–6.

17. McSharry DG, Ryan S, Calverley P, et al. Sleep quality in chronic obstructive pulmonary disease. Respirology 2012;17(7):1119–24.

18. McNicholas WT. Impact of sleep on ventilation and gas exchange in chronic lung disease. Monaldi Arch Chest Dis 2003;59(3):212–5.

19. Zanchet RC, Viegas CA. Nocturnal desaturation: predictors and the effect on sleep patterns in patients with chronic obstructive pulmonary disease and concomitant mild daytime hypoxemia. J Bras Pneumol 2006;32(3):207–12.

20. Li SQ, Sun XW, Zhang L, et al. Impact of insomnia and obstructive sleep apnea on the risk of acute exacerbation of chronic obstructive pulmonary disease. Sleep Med Rev 2021;58:101444.

21. Hong YD, Onukwugha E, Slejko JF. The economic burden of Comorbid obstructive sleep apnea among patients with chronic obstructive pulmonary disease. J Manag Care Spec Pharm 2020;26(10):1353–62.

22. McNicholas WT. Does associated chronic obstructive pulmonary disease increase morbidity and mortality in obstructive sleep apnea? Ann Am Thorac Soc 2019;16(1):50–3.

23. Vanfleteren LE, Beghe B, Andersson A, et al. Multimorbidity in COPD, does sleep matter? Eur J Intern Med 2020;73:7–15.

24. Eckert DJ, Butler JE. Respiratory physiology: understanding the control of ventilation. In: Kryger MH, Roth T, Dement WC, editors. Principles and practice of sleep medicine. 6th edition. Philadelphia (PA): Elsevier; 2017. p. p167–73.

25. Boing S, Randerath WJ. Chronic hypoventilation syndromes and sleep-related hypoventilation. J Thorac Dis 2015;7(8):1273–85.

26. Sowho M, Amatoury J, Kirkness JP, et al. Sleep and respiratory physiology in adults. Clin Chest Med 2014;35(3):469–81.

27. Douglas NJ, White DP, Weil JV, et al. Hypercapnic ventilatory response in sleeping adults. Am Rev Respir Dis 1982;126(5):758–62.

28. Bulow K. Respiration and wakefulness in man. Acta Physiol Scand Suppl 1963;209:1–110.

29. Hedemark LL, Kronenberg RS. Ventilatory and heart rate responses to hypoxia and hypercapnia during sleep in adults. J Appl Physiol Respir Environ Exerc Physiol 1982;53(2):307–12.

30. White DP, Douglas NJ, Pickett CK, et al. Hypoxic ventilatory response during sleep in normal premenopausal women. Am Rev Respir Dis 1982;126(3):530–3.

31. Wheatley JR, White DP. The influence of sleep on pharyngeal reflexes. Sleep 1993;16(8 Suppl):S87–9.

32. Tangel DJ, Mezzanotte WS, White DP. Influence of sleep on tensor palatini EMG and upper airway resistance in normal men. J Appl Physiol (1985) 1991;70(6):2574–81.

33. Hudgel DW, Devadatta P. Decrease in functional residual capacity during sleep in normal humans.

J Appl Physiol Respir Environ Exerc Physiol 1984; 57(5):1319–22.

34. Saper CB, Scammell TE, Lu J. Hypothalamic regulation of sleep and circadian rhythms. Nature 2005; 437(7063):1257–63.

35. McNicholas WT, Hansson D, Schiza S, et al. Sleep in chronic respiratory disease: COPD and hypoventilation disorders. Eur Respir Rev 2019; 28(153):190064.

36. Trask CH, Cree EM. Oximeter studies on patients with chronic obstructive emphysema, awake and during sleep. N Engl J Med 1962;266:639–42.

37. Lange P, Marott JL, Vestbo J, et al. Prevalence of night-time dyspnoea in COPD and its implications for prognosis. Eur Respir J 2014;43(6):1590–8.

38. McNicholas WT. Impact of sleep in COPD. Chest 2000;117(2 Suppl):48s–53s.

39. Becker HF, Piper AJ, Flynn WE, et al. Breathing during sleep in patients with nocturnal desaturation. Am J Respir Crit Care Med 1999;159(1):112–8.

40. Johnson MW, Remmers JE. Accessory muscle activity during sleep in chronic obstructive pulmonary disease. J Appl Physiol Respir Environ Exerc Physiol 1984;57(4):1011–7.

41. McNicholas WT, Verbraecken J, Marin JM. Sleep disorders in COPD: the forgotten dimension. Eur Respir Rev 2013;22(129):365–75.

42. O'Donnell DE, Webb KA. The major limitation to exercise performance in COPD is dynamic hyperinflation. J Appl Physiol (1985) 2008;105(2):753–5 [discussion: 755–7].

43. Motley HL. The effects of slow deep breathing on the blood gas exchange in emphysema. Am Rev Respir Dis 1963;88:484–92.

44. Ingram RH Jr, Schilder DP. Effect of pursed lips expiration on the pulmonary pressure-flow relationship in obstructive lung disease. Am Rev Respir Dis 1967;96(3):381–8.

45. Catterall JR, Calverley PM, MacNee W, et al. Mechanism of transient nocturnal hypoxemia in hypoxic chronic bronchitis and emphysema. J Appl Physiol (1985) 1985;59(6):1698–703.

46. Hudgel DW, Martin RJ, Capehart M, et al. Contribution of hypoventilation to sleep oxygen desaturation in chronic obstructive pulmonary disease. J Appl Physiol Respir Environ Exerc Physiol 1983;55(3): 669–77.

47. Mulloy E, Fitzpatrick M, Bourke S, et al. Oxygen desaturation during sleep and exercise in patients with severe chronic obstructive pulmonary disease. Respir Med 1995;89(3):193–8.

48. Chaouat A, Weitzenblum E, Kessler R, et al. Sleep-related O2 desaturation and daytime pulmonary haemodynamics in COPD patients with mild hypoxaemia. Eur Respir J 1997;10(8):1730–5.

49. Patel SR. Obstructive sleep apnea. Ann Intern Med 2019;171(11):Itc81–96.

50. Peppard PE, Young T, Barnet JH, et al. Increased prevalence of sleep-disordered breathing in adults. Am J Epidemiol 2013;177(9):1006–14.

51. Young T, Palta M, Dempsey J, et al. The occurrence of sleep-disordered breathing among middle-aged adults. N Engl J Med 1993;328(17): 1230–5.

52. Sanders MH, Newman AB, Haggerty CL, et al. Sleep and sleep-disordered breathing in adults with predominantly mild obstructive airway disease. Am J Respir Crit Care Med 2003;167(1): 7–14.

53. Flenley DC. Sleep in chronic obstructive lung disease. Clin Chest Med 1985;6(4):651–61.

54. Bednarek M, Plywaczewski R, Jonczak L, et al. There is no relationship between chronic obstructive pulmonary disease and obstructive sleep apnea syndrome: a population study. Respiration 2005;72(2):142–9.

55. Nattusami L, Hadda V, Khilnani GC, et al. Co-existing obstructive sleep apnea among patients with chronic obstructive pulmonary disease. Lung India 2021;38(1):12–7.

56. Shawon MS, Perret JL, Senaratna CV, et al. Current evidence on prevalence and clinical outcomes of co-morbid obstructive sleep apnea and chronic obstructive pulmonary disease: a systematic review. Sleep Med Rev 2017;32:58–68.

57. Stanchina ML, Welicky LM, Donat W, et al. Impact of CPAP use and age on mortality in patients with combined COPD and obstructive sleep apnea: the overlap syndrome. J Clin Sleep Med 2013; 9(8):767–72.

58. Chaouat A, Weitzenblum E, Krieger J, et al. Association of chronic obstructive pulmonary disease and sleep apnea syndrome. Am J Respir Crit Care Med 1995;151(1):82–6.

59. Greenberg-Dotan S, Reuveni H, Tal A, et al. Increased prevalence of obstructive lung disease in patients with obstructive sleep apnea. Sleep Breath 2014;18(1):69–75.

60. Shiina K, Tomiyama H, Takata Y, et al. Overlap syndrome: additive effects of COPD on the cardiovascular damages in patients with OSA. Respir Med 2012;106(9):1335–41.

61. Larsson LG, Lindberg A, Franklin KA, et al. Obstructive Lung Disease in Northern Sweden S. Obstructive sleep apnoea syndrome is common in subjects with chronic bronchitis. Report from the Obstructive Lung Disease in Northern Sweden studies. Respiration 2001;68(3):250–5.

62. Machado MC, Vollmer WM, Togeiro SM, et al. CPAP and survival in moderate-to-severe obstructive sleep apnoea syndrome and hypoxaemic COPD. Eur Respir J 2010;35(1):132–7.

63. Orr JE, Schmickl CN, Edwards BA, et al. Pathogenesis of obstructive sleep apnea in individuals with

the COPD + OSA Overlap syndrome versus OSA alone. Physiol Rep 2020;8(3):e14371.

64. Prasad B, Nyenhuis SM, Imayama I, et al. Asthma and obstructive sleep apnea overlap: what has the evidence taught us? Am J Respir Crit Care Med 2020;201(11):1345–57.

65. Maselli DJ, Hanania NA. Asthma COPD overlap: impact of associated comorbidities. Pulm Pharmacol Ther 2018;52:27–31.

66. Adler D, Bailly S, Benmerad M, et al. Clinical presentation and comorbidities of obstructive sleep apnea-COPD overlap syndrome. PLoS One 2020; 15(7):e0235331.

67. Diomidous M, Marios N, Zikos D, et al. The syndrome of sleep apnea in the Elderly suffering from COPD and live in the County of Attica, Greece. Mater Sociomed 2012;24(4):227–31.

68. O'Brien A, Whitman K. Lack of benefit of continuous positive airway pressure on lung function in patients with overlap syndrome. Lung 2005; 183(6):389–404.

69. Kuvat N, Tanriverdi H, Armutcu F. The relationship between obstructive sleep apnea syndrome and obesity: a new perspective on the pathogenesis in terms of organ crosstalk. Clin Respir J 2020; 14(7):595–604.

70. Deegan PC, McNicholas WT. Pathophysiology of obstructive sleep apnoea. Eur Respir J 1995;8(7): 1161–78.

71. Steveling EH, Clarenbach CF, Miedinger D, et al. Predictors of the overlap syndrome and its association with comorbidities in patients with chronic obstructive pulmonary disease. Respiration 2014; 88(6):451–7.

72. McNicholas WT. COPD-OSA overlap syndrome: Evolving evidence regarding Epidemiology, clinical consequences, and management. Chest 2017; 152(6):1318–26.

73. Biselli P, Grossman PR, Kirkness JP, et al. The effect of increased lung volume in chronic obstructive pulmonary disease on upper airway obstruction during sleep. J Appl Physiol (1985) 2015;119(3):266–71.

74. McNicholas WT. Chronic obstructive pulmonary disease and obstructive sleep apnea: overlaps in pathophysiology, systemic inflammation, and cardiovascular disease. Am J Respir Crit Care Med 2009;180(8):692–700.

75. Wetter DW, Young TB, Bidwell TR, et al. Smoking as a risk factor for sleep-disordered breathing. Arch Intern Med 1994;154(19):2219–24.

76. Redolfi S, Yumino D, Ruttanaumpawan P, et al. Relationship between overnight rostral fluid shift and Obstructive Sleep Apnea in nonobese men. Am J Respir Crit Care Med 2009;179(3):241–6.

77. Takabatake N, Nakamura H, Abe S, et al. The relationship between chronic hypoxemia and

activation of the tumor necrosis factor-alpha system in patients with chronic obstructive pulmonary disease. Am J Respir Crit Care Med 2000;161(4 Pt 1):1179–84.

78. Tirlapur VG, Mir MA. Nocturnal hypoxemia and associated electrocardiographic changes in patients with chronic obstructive airways disease. N Engl J Med 1982;306(3):125–30.

79. Hawryłkiewicz I, Sliwiński P, Górecka D, et al. Pulmonary haemodynamics in patients with OSAS or an overlap syndrome. Monaldi Arch Chest Dis 2004;61(3):148–52.

80. Ordronneau J, Chollet S, Nogues B, et al. [Sleep apnea syndrome in intensive care]. Rev Mal Respir 1994;11(1):51–5.

81. Jaoude P, El-Solh AA. Predictive factors for COPD exacerbations and mortality in patients with overlap syndrome. Clin Respir J 2019;13(10):643–51.

82. Donovan LM, Feemster LC, Udris EM, et al. Poor outcomes among patients with chronic obstructive pulmonary disease with higher risk for undiagnosed obstructive sleep apnea in the LOTT cohort. J Clin Sleep Med 2019;15(1):71–7.

83. Marin JM, Soriano JB, Carrizo SJ, et al. Outcomes in patients with chronic obstructive pulmonary disease and obstructive sleep apnea: the overlap syndrome. Am J Respir Crit Care Med 2010;182(3): 325–31.

84. Lavie P, Herer P, Lavie L. Mortality risk factors in sleep apnoea: a matched case-control study. J Sleep Res 2007;16(1):128–34.

85. Faria AC, da Costa CH, Rufino R. Sleep apnea clinical score, Berlin questionnaire, or Epworth sleepiness scale: which is the best obstructive sleep apnea predictor in patients with COPD? Int J Gen Med 2015;8:275–81.

86. Soler X, Liao SY, Marin JM, et al. Age, gender, neck circumference, and Epworth sleepiness scale do not predict obstructive sleep apnea (OSA) in moderate to severe chronic obstructive pulmonary disease (COPD): the challenge to predict OSA in advanced COPD. PLoS One 2017;12(5):e0177289.

87. Lajoie AC, Sériès F, Bernard S, et al. Reliability of home nocturnal oximetry in the diagnosis of overlap syndrome in COPD. Respiration 2020;99(2):132–9.

88. Scott AS, Baltzan MA, Wolkove N. Examination of pulse oximetry tracings to detect obstructive sleep apnea in patients with advanced chronic obstructive pulmonary disease. Can Respir J 2014;21(3): 171–5.

89. Kapur VK, Auckley DH, Chowdhuri S, et al. Clinical practice guideline for diagnostic testing for adult obstructive sleep apnea: an american academy of sleep medicine clinical practice guideline. J Clin Sleep Med 2017;13(3):479–504.

90. Oliveira MG, Nery LE, Santos-Silva R, et al. Is portable monitoring accurate in the diagnosis of

obstructive sleep apnea syndrome in chronic pulmonary obstructive disease? Sleep Med 2012; 13(8):1033–8.

91. Celli BR, MacNee W, Agusti A, et al. Standards for the diagnosis and treatment of patients with COPD: a summary of the ATS/ERS position paper. Eur Respir J 2004;23(6):932–46.

92. Alford NJ, Fletcher EC, Nickeson D. Acute oxygen in patients with sleep apnea and COPD. Chest 1986;89(1):30–8.

93. Zeineddine S, Rowley JA, Chowdhuri S. Oxygen therapy in sleep-disordered breathing. Chest 2021;160(2):701–17.

94. Konikkara J, Tavella R, Willes L, et al. Early recognition of obstructive sleep apnea in patients hospitalized with COPD exacerbation is associated with reduced readmission. Hosp Pract (1995) 2016; 44(1):41–7.

95. de Miguel J, Cabello J, Sanchez-Alarcos JM, et al. Long-term effects of treatment with nasal continuous positive airway pressure on lung function in patients with overlap syndrome. Sleep Breath 2002;6(1):3–10.

96. Mansfield D, Naughton MT. Effects of continuous positive airway pressure on lung function in patients with chronic obstructive pulmonary disease and sleep disordered breathing. Respirology 1999;4(4):365–70.

97. McDonald CF, Whyte K, Jenkins S, et al. Clinical practice guideline on adult domiciliary oxygen therapy: Executive summary from the thoracic society of Australia and New Zealand. Respirology 2016; 21(1):76–8.

98. Levi-Valensi P, Weitzenblum E, Rida Z, et al. Sleep-related oxygen desaturation and daytime pulmonary haemodynamics in COPD patients. Eur Respir J 1992;5(3):301–7.

99. Lacasse Y, Series F, Vujovic-Zotovic N, et al. Evaluating nocturnal oxygen desaturation in COPD–revised. Respir Med 2011;105(9):1331–7.

100. Vos PJ, Folgering HT, van Herwaarden CL. Predictors for nocturnal hypoxaemia (mean SaO2 < 90%) in normoxic and mildly hypoxic patients with COPD. Eur Respir J 1995;8(1):74–7.

101. Fletcher EC, Miller J, Divine GW, et al. Nocturnal oxyhemoglobin desaturation in COPD patients with arterial oxygen tensions above 60 mm Hg. Chest 1987;92(4):604–8.

102. Hardinge M, Annandale J, Bourne S, et al. British Thoracic Society guidelines for home oxygen use in adults. Thorax 2015;70(Suppl 1):i1–43.

103. Jacobs SS, Krishnan JA, Lederer DJ, et al. Home oxygen therapy for adults with chronic lung disease. an official american thoracic society clinical practice guideline. Am J Respir Crit Care Med 2020;202(10):e121–41.

104. Sliwiński P, Lagosz M, Górecka D, et al. The adequacy of oxygenation in COPD patients undergoing long-term oxygen therapy assessed by pulse oximetry at home. Eur Respir J 1994; 7(2):274–8.

105. Zhu Z, Barnette RK, Fussell KM, et al. Continuous oxygen monitoring–a better way to prescribe long-term oxygen therapy. Respir Med 2005; 99(11):1386–92.

106. Morrison D, Skwarski KM, MacNee W. The adequacy of oxygenation in patients with hypoxic chronic obstructive pulmonary disease treated with long-term domiciliary oxygen. Respir Med 1997;91(5):287–91.

107. Continuous or nocturnal oxygen therapy in hypoxemic chronic obstructive lung disease: a clinical trial. Nocturnal Oxygen Therapy Trial Group. Ann Intern Med 1980;93(3):391–8.

108. Lewis CA, Fergusson W, Eaton T, et al. Isolated nocturnal desaturation in COPD: prevalence and impact on quality of life and sleep. Thorax 2009; 64(2):133–8.

109. Sergi M, Rizzi M, Andreoli A, et al. Are COPD patients with nocturnal REM sleep-related desaturations more prone to developing chronic respiratory failure requiring long-term oxygen therapy? Respiration 2002;69(2):117–22.

110. Fletcher EC, Luckett RA, Miller T, et al. Pulmonary vascular hemodynamics in chronic lung disease patients with and without oxyhemoglobin desaturation during sleep. Chest 1989;95(4):757–64.

111. Fletcher EC, Luckett RA, Goodnight-White S, et al. A double-blind trial of nocturnal supplemental oxygen for sleep desaturation in patients with chronic obstructive pulmonary disease and a daytime PaO2 above 60 mm Hg. Am Rev Respir Dis 1992;145(5):1070–6.

112. Fletcher EC, Donner CF, Midgren B, et al. Survival in COPD patients with a daytime PaO2 greater than 60 mm Hg with and without nocturnal oxyhemoglobin desaturation. Chest 1992;101(3): 649–55.

113. 0Lacasse Y, Series F, Martin S, et al. Nocturnal oxygen therapy in patients with chronic obstructive pulmonary disease: a survey of Canadian respirologists. Can Respir J 2007;14(6):343–8.

114. Macrea MM, Owens RL, Martin T, et al. The effect of isolated nocturnal oxygen desaturations on serum hs-CRP and IL-6 in patients with chronic obstructive pulmonary disease. Clin Respir J 2019;13(2): 120–4.

115. Alexandre F, Heraud N, Varray A. Is nocturnal desaturation a trigger for neuronal damage in chronic obstructive pulmonary disease? Med Hypotheses 2015;84(1):25–30.

116. Chaouat A, Weitzenblum E, Kessler R, et al. A randomized trial of nocturnal oxygen therapy in chronic obstructive pulmonary disease patients. Eur Respir J 1999;14(5):1002–8.

117. Orth M, Walther JW, Yalzin S, et al. [Influence of nocturnal oxygen therapy on quality of life in patients with COPD and isolated sleep-related hypoxemia: a prospective, placebo-controlled cross-over trial]. Pneumologie 2008;62(1):11–6.

118. Lacasse Y, Sériès F, Corbeil F, et al. Randomized trial of nocturnal oxygen in chronic obstructive pulmonary disease. N Engl J Med 2020;383(12): 1129–38.

119. Tan L, Latshang TD, Aeschbacher SS, et al. Effect of nocturnal oxygen therapy on nocturnal hypoxemia and sleep apnea among patients with chronic obstructive pulmonary disease traveling to 2048 meters: a randomized clinical trial. JAMA Netw Open 2020;3(6):e207940.

120. O'Donoghue FJ, Catcheside PG, Ellis EE, et al. Sleep hypoventilation in hypercapnic chronic obstructive pulmonary disease: prevalence and associated factors. Eur Respir J 2003;21(6):977–84.

121. Osadnik CR, Tee VS, Carson-Chahhoud KV, et al. Non-invasive ventilation for the management of acute hypercapnic respiratory failure due to exacerbation of chronic obstructive pulmonary disease. Cochrane Database Syst Rev 2017;7(7): Cd004104.

122. Foucher P, Baudouin N, Merati M, et al. Relative survival analysis of 252 patients with COPD receiving long-term oxygen therapy. Chest 1998; 113(6):1580–7.

123. Ahmadi Z, Bornefalk-Hermansson A, Franklin KA, et al. Hypo- and hypercapnia predict mortality in oxygen-dependent chronic obstructive pulmonary disease: a population-based prospective study. Respir Res 2014;15(1):30.

124. Budweiser S, Heinemann F, Fischer W, et al. Long-term reduction of hyperinflation in stable COPD by non-invasive nocturnal home ventilation. Respir Med 2005;99(8):976–84.

125. Clinical indications for noninvasive positive pressure ventilation in chronic respiratory failure due to restrictive lung disease, COPD, and nocturnal hypoventilation–a consensus conference report. Chest 1999;116(2):521–34.

126. Nickol AH, Hart N, Hopkinson NS, et al. Mechanisms of improvement of respiratory failure in patients with COPD treated with NIV. Int J Chron Obstruct Pulmon Dis 2008;3(3):453–62.

127. Macrea M, Oczkowski S, Rochwerg B, et al. Long-term noninvasive ventilation in chronic stable hypercapnic chronic obstructive pulmonary disease. an official American Thoracic Society Clinical Practice Guideline. Am J Respir Crit Care Med 2020; 202(4):e74–87.

128. Ergan B, Oczkowski S, Rochwerg B, et al. European Respiratory Society guidelines on long-term home non-invasive ventilation for management of COPD. Eur Respir J 2019;54(3):1901003.

Sleep and Obesity

Ji Hyun Lee, MD*, Jahyeon Cho, MD

KEYWORDS

- Sleep • OSA • Appetite • Leptin • Ghrelin • Obesity

KEY POINTS

- Poor sleep leads to inadequate appetite control and obesity deteriorates sleep quality.
- Sleep deprivation either quality or quantity, makes people tired and fatigue, affecting appetite, and ultimately leading to obesity.
- Delayed sleep phase is associated not only insomnia symptom but also nocturnal binge eating.
- Overweight people can develop sleep complaints that may deteriorate the quality of sleep such as OSA.
- Sleep and obesity have mutual influence and further exacerbate the other.

INTRODUCTION

Daytime fatigue or excessive daytime sleepiness are common sequelae of disturbed nocturnal sleep seen in certain conditions such as obstructive sleep apnea (OSA). We witnessed the advances in sleep science after the discovery of OSA and obesity hypoventilation syndrome (OHS), which is often referred to as the "Pickwickian syndrome." Obesity and male gender were known risk factors for sleep disorders as early as the 1800s.

Recent interest in obesity developed when the association between short sleep time and increased body mass index (BMI) was published in 2002.[1] Shortly after, in 2004, scientific investigation found the association of leptin and ghrelin with sleep.[2,3] Since then, there have been thousands of research on sleep and obesity from the molecular level, epidemiologic data, observational studies, and experimental studies, in both animals and humans. Nowadays, people value the importance of sleep quantity and quality in weight control in order to maintain a healthier lifestyle.

In the past, eating voraciously at night was only perceived as a psychological representation of losing self-control. This changed after the impact of the circadian sleep-wake cycle on appetite control started to receive attention.

In a study conducted in 2021, researchers found that not only is sleep duration important, the timing of sleep was also significant.[4]

Here, we will discuss the impact of sleep on appetite and obesity, and in turn, the influence of weight or body composition on sleep and sleep disorders.

MOLECULAR PATHOLOGY
Leptin and Ghrelin

Leptin and ghrelin are two important hormones that help maintain energy balance. Leptin is known as the "appetite suppressor" and is synthesized in adipose tissue. Its direct relationship with the amount of body fat was first reported in 1994.[5] Early reports of leptin injections in leptin-deficient patients with childhood obesity showed improved appetite and energy expenditure.[6] However, in non–leptin-deficient obese patients, when leptin was directly administered, it did not improve obesity.[7] It was later determined that this was due to leptin resistance, which was identified as the major pathology leading to obesity. To date, the exact mechanism of leptin resistance remains unclear.

Ghrelin increases food intake by increasing the appetite. It is released mainly in the stomach and is presumed to signal hunger to the brain. The level of ghrelin in the blood increases when the energy is low, such as during fasting or starvation. Ghrelin levels rapidly increase after food intake. Its secretion is also affected by sleep, such as during sleep deprivation.

Studies have revealed an association between sleep time and these appetite-regulating

Department of Psychiatry, Dream Sleep Clinic, 107, Dosandaero, Gangnamgu, Seoul, South Korea
* Corresponding author.
E-mail address: lee.jihyun.md@gmail.com

Sleep Med Clin 17 (2022) 111–116
https://doi.org/10.1016/j.jsmc.2021.10.009
1556-407X/22/© 2021 Elsevier Inc. All rights reserved.

sleep.theclinics.com

hormones. In 2004, Spiegel and colleagues found that sleep restriction is associated with reduction of leptin by 18% and elevation of ghrelin by 24%. He also showed that sleep restriction causes individuals to seek calorie-dense food such as high carbohydrate food.[3] Studies on sleep restriction and leptin/ghrelin were subsequently made, and a recent meta-analysis published in 2020 suggested that short sleep duration was associated with increased ghrelin levels, whereas sleep deprivation significantly affected both leptin and ghrelin levels.[8]

Role of Orexin in Weight Control

Hypocretin (orexin) was first identified by two different groups in 1998. It is known to regulate sleep, wakefulness, and appetite. Hypocretin is now thought to be a major modulator in the brain, affecting other neurotransmitters, such as acetylcholine, norepinephrine, histamine, and serotonin. It is also presumed to regulate behavior in times of physiologic needs and body reaction to threats; however, its main role is just beginning to be understood.

One of its main roles is to regulate sleep and wakefulness. It was found that the hypocretin neurons are completely destroyed in narcolepsy. Decreased level or absence of hypocretin in the cerebrospinal fluid is found in almost all the patients with narcolepsy type I. The BMI of patients with narcolepsy is found to be significantly higher than that in non-narcolepsy patients.[9,10] Although the mechanism is not fully understood, it is proposed that orexin co-localization in the lateral hypothalamus plays a role in comorbid narcolepsy and obesity.

Developmental explanation of short sleep and weight gain in children and adolescents.

In 1996, over 8000 children aged 6 to 7 years were investigated to determine the relationship between sleep time and weight in Toyama prefecture, Japan. Researchers have found that there is a dose-response relationship between late bedtimes, short sleep hours, and childhood obesity.[11] Since then, thousands of articles have been published. In a recent meta-analysis of prospective cohort studies published in 2021, researchers found that there is a dose-response relationship between sleep time and obesity in children, especially within 3 to 13 years of age.[12] This showed that childhood weight gain is associated with public health issues, including negative psychological and physical consequences. Children with short sleep duration can also develop worse mood symptoms, such as depression, attention problems, and eating disorders.[13]

The physical complications associated with obesity include childhood diabetes mellitus, dyslipidemia, insulin resistance, asthma, polycystic ovarian syndrome, and elevated blood pressure.[14,15] Obese children may develop OSA, further causing sleep fragmentation, which in turn causes weight control problems.

Children with obesity tend to remain obese when they grow up. Both genetic and environmental factors influence the parenting and eating habits in families. Short sleep duration and obesity link in children also has genetic background, and genes like "Suz12 target genes," or "PAX3-FOXO1 target genes" were suggested.[16] Short sleep duration in the early stage of life is associated with poor weight control and further deteriorates the quality of life.

Epidemiologic Data Explaining Sleep Duration and Weight Control

Experimental studies—sleep deprivation test
The sleep deprivation test was performed in late 1960 by Kuhn and colleagues. Scientists aimed to observe the various impacts of partial or total sleep deprivation, especially on metabolism. They saw an increase in the appetite (20% of subjective food consumption), as well as weight gain (+0.4 kg) over 4 nights of 5.5 h of sleep (partial sleep deprivation group). Notably, an increase in the appetite was observed in the evening.[17,18] Nowadays in dealing with obese patients, a routine evaluation of sleep time has become the standard of practice.

Case-Control Observational Studies
A study of 327 obese children and 704 controls at the age of 5 revealed that short nocturnal sleep is the only variable associated with obesity (adjusted odds ratio = 1.4), not snack eating habits or television watching.[19] There is a meta-analysis of 45 studies showing increased risk of obesity among short sleepers in children and adults.[20] It is said that children are more vulnerable than adults, whereas young adults are prone to develop obesity than mid-life and late-life adults.[21]

Longitudinal Epidemiologic Studies
In the Penn State Cohort with a follow-up period of 7.5 years, it revealed that nonobese adults with subjective short sleep duration were at risk of developing obesity. Those with poor sleep who developed obesity initially showed the shortest sleep duration and the highest level of emotional stress at baseline. Subjective short sleep duration ($\leq$5 h) is associated with increased incident obesity with an odds ratio of 2.18.[22] CARDIA sleep study also[23] confirms that short sleep duration is associated with developing obesity in the long term.

SLEEP DISORDERS AND OBESITY
OSA and obesity

Obesity and OSA have a mutual relationship. Obesity is a well-known risk factor for OSA. As a patient becomes obese, the upper airway is almost always affected. During breathing, the upper airway is maintained patent with the balance of intraluminal negative pressure from the diaphragm during inspiration and extraluminal pressure surrounding the upper airway. The soft tissue affecting the airway includes muscles, such as the genioglossus and tensor palatini, adipose tissue surrounding the airway, and bony structures. Obesity negatively affects the airway by increasing fat deposition inside and outside of the muscles surrounding the airway and increasing collapsibility of the airway. Central obesity due to abdominal fat also affects the upper airway.

OSA in turn is known to aggravate obesity. OSA patients complain of excessive daytime sleepiness, and as a result, significantly diminishing their physical activity.[24,25] It is postulated that use of electronic devices and marked decrease in physical activity, as a result of a shift to indoor life, contribute to low physical activity.

Low sleep quality and fragmented nocturnal sleep contribute to diminished leptin levels, which is associated with obesity in patients with OSA.

There are controversies regarding whether therapeutic interventions, such as continuous positive airway pressure (CPAP), lead to increased physical activity.[26,27] CPAP therapy is presumed to reduce weight as it may stabilize the metabolism of the body and nocturnal sleep; however, CPAP or other therapeutic interventions did not facilitate significant changes in either weight or basal metabolic rate (BMR). CPAP may contribute to weight gain, contrary to our expectations.[28,29] There is a large-scale randomized controlled study to examine the effect of CPAP in patients with OSA called the Apnea Positive Pressure Long-term Efficacy Study (APPLES), which contradicts the common presumption that CPAP-compliant users experienced weight gain instead of weight loss. Notably, the patient group that used CPAP for more than 4 hours per night out of 70% of nights (CPAP-compliant) showed more weight gain than the sham CPAP (CPAP with a pressure of 4 cm H_2O) or CPAP noncompliant groups. Moreover, the authors reported a dose-response relationship between the hours of adherence and amount of weight gained.

Likewise, adenotonsillectomy for OSA in overweight children resulted in weight gain, identical to the effect of CPAP on weight change in the adult OSA group.[30] Hence, therapeutic interventions for OSA can be thought to reduce energy consumption.

Energy expenditure, which is the sum of the BMR (the amount of energy expended while at complete rest), thermic effect of food (the energy required to digest and absorb food), and energy expended in physical activity, changes in patients with OSA after treatment. The OSA patients need a higher energy expenditure (EE) in the 24-h resting state and during sleep than those without OSA. Additional work may be needed to breathe, as observed throughout the night in chronic obstructive lung disease patients.[31,32] Sympathetic hyperexcitation in response to hypoxemia and/or arousals at the end of apnea/hypopnea events, resulting in fragmented sleep, may also contribute to higher EE in OSA patients.[33]

The endless cycle of the effects of OSA on obesity, and vice versa, is not easy to stop. Clinicians should not depend on the physiologic effects of CPAP in OSA patients to control their weight. Lifestyle modification should be included in the treatment protocol of patients with OSA. The introduction of lifestyle and dietary modifications on top of standard CPAP therapy would provide the best results for OSA patients in the long run.[34,35]

Obesity Hypoventilation Syndrome

OHS is defined as a combination of obesity (BMI $\geq$ 30 kg/m^2), sleep-disordered breathing, and daytime hypercapnia (Paco$_2$ $\geq$ 45 mm Hg at sea level) in the absence of an alternative neuromuscular, metabolic, or mechanical explanation for hypercapnia. It is usually diagnosed late when chronic respiratory failure results in sharp deterioration, the so-called acute-on-chronic hypercapnic respiratory failure. The diagnosis is usually made in the fifties and sixties age group.

Nearly 90% of patients with OHS have sleep apnea and 70% have severe OSA. When OSA is present along with OHS, a diagnosis of both OSA and OHS should be made.[36]

Room air arterial blood gas analysis is a definitive diagnostic test for daytime hypercapnia. If not, a daytime serum bicarbonate level (<27 mEq/L) should be measured to rule out daytime hypercapnia. If this method is not available, low oxygen level measured by pulse oximetry during the daytime can be helpful. However, clinicians should know that there are other reasons for daytime hypoxemia and, ultimately, daytime hypercapnia is needed to make a firm diagnosis.[37]

Positive airway pressure (PAP) therapy is the main treatment method for patients with OHS.

Many patients respond to CPAP or bilevel PAP with improvement in daytime $Paco_2$; however, complete resolution of daytime hypercapnia may not be evident.

Narcolepsy and Obesity

As previously described, the co-location of orexin/hypocretin neurons in the lateral hypothalamus is considered as the main pathology for narcolepsy-associated obesity. People with narcolepsy who do not eat more than average, yet still gain weight. It is proposed that this sudden dramatic weight gain is associated with lower body metabolism, or direct effect of hypocretin.[10] BMI seems unrelated to the disease severity and medication status.[9] Longitudinal follow-up study of childhood narcolepsy type I patients for 36 months showed more propensity to become obese (38.46%) and overweight (26.15%). Authors suggest this is related to decreased energy expenditure especially in the early stage of disease course, which gets less prominent later on.[38] So, it is important to emphasize role of exercise in childhood narcolepsy, not worrying about aggravating cataplectic symptoms.[39]

Pathophysiologically, obesity associated with orexin (OX) depletion in OX-null mice is linked to brown-fat hypoactivity, which leads to dampening of energy expenditure. Further research is needed to see the causal relationship between narcolepsy and obesity.[40]

Circadian Rhythm and Appetite

The so-called social jet lag group showed an increased appetite for calorie-dense food. Even without sleep deprivation, changing sleep time is associated with appetite change. Individuals in the social jet lag group showed later mealtimes for lunch and dinner. Therefore, the quality and quantity of sleep, as well as the circadian timing, affect the appetite and food intake.[4] Circadian shift to a later bedtime, with developmentally decreasing sleep drive power as well as psychosocial factors such as extracurricular activities, homework, electronic device usage, easier access to caffeinated beverages may contribute to aggravating sleep phase change in teenagers. People with delayed sleep phase showed even less ability to compensate for previous sleep loss.[41]

Circadian rhythm sleep disorders and shift workers are prone to obesity. A recent meta-analysis showed that night shift workers have an increased risk of obesity/overweight.[42] Permanent night workers are observed to have 29% higher risk than rotating shift workers (odds ratio 1.43 vs 1.14).[43] Short duration and poor quality of sleep are considered to increase the risk of developing obesity. Timing of food intake is important, for inappropriate circadian meal timing, or food intake during biological nights, and also contributes to obesity.[44]

Sleep Debt and Obesity

Public awareness about the fact that total sleep time is decreased because of industrial and cultural development, and that shift work is harmful to health are increased. A recent review shows that there is not a huge change in the sleep duration over the past 50+ decades, both subjectively and objectively.[45]

It should be noted that, in this review, it was shown that the total sleep time of children and adolescents had decreased as well. Sleep debt in the early stages of life has a significant impact on the physical, psychological, and developmental points of view.

In 1999, the metabolic and endocrinological impact of short sleep duration was suggested; sleeping less than 6 hours is associated with increased morbidity specifically obesity, type 2 diabetes, cardiovascular disease, and risk of accidents. Short sleep duration is consistently associated with increased BMI as seen in many epidemiologic studies and experiments, especially in children and adolescence.[46,47]

DISCUSSION

Sleep and obesity share a mutual relationship in which they aggravate each other. Short sleep duration is associated with leptin resistance and ghrelin secretion, resulting in uncontrollable appetite. Diseases that affect the quality of sleep also have a bad influence on weight control. Poor meal timing could worsen the irregularity of sleep thereby making it difficult to regulate food choices and appetite. Unfortunately, neither weekend sleep nor naps compensate for sleep debt.

A large prospective epidemiologic study is still needed to further confirm gender difference and to find ways to minimize the impact of bright light exposure from gadgets and change in sleep schedules, especially in adolescence.

Obesity also disturbs sleep in turn, causing further sleep fragmentation and deterioration. Poor quality of sleep impacts our daily level of alertness, power to concentrate, and energy. Physical and psychological complications from poor sleep associated with obesity are usually chronic causing debilitating consequences.

CLINICS CARE POINTS

- Short sleep duration increases the risk of developing obesity in young children, adolescence, and adults. Epidemiologic data, as well as investigation on leptin, ghrelin, and orexin neuropeptide, show the impact of sleep loss on weight control.

- Sleep disorders, like OSA result in sleep fragmentation and obesity.

- Management of OSA using CPAP does not solve already problematic weight gain without concomitant lifestyle change.

DISCLOSURE

The authors have nothing to disclose.

REFERENCES

1. Kripke DF, Garfinkel L, Wingard DL, et al. Mortality associated with sleep duration and insomnia. Arch Gen Psychiatry 2002;59(2):131–6.
2. Taheri S, Lin L, Austin D, et al. Short sleep duration is associated with reduced leptin, elevated ghrelin, and increased body mass index. Plos Med 2004; 1(3):e62.
3. Spiegel K, Tasali E, Penev P, et al. Brief communication: sleep curtailment in healthy young men is associated with decreased leptin levels, elevated ghrelin levels, and increased hunger and appetite. Ann Intern Med 2004;141(11):846–50.
4. Suikki T, Maukonen M, Partonen T, et al. Association between social jet lag, quality of diet and obesity by diurnal preference in Finnish adult population. Chronobiol Int 2021;38(5):720–31.
5. Zhang Y, Proenca R, Maffei M, et al. Positional cloning of the mouse obese gene and its human homologue. Nature 1994;372:425–32.
6. Farooqi IS, Jebb SA, Langmack G, et al. Effects of recombinant leptin therapy in a child with congenital leptin deficiency. N Engl J Med 1999;341(12): 879–84.
7. Woods SC, Schwartz MW, Baskin DG, et al. Food intake and the regulation of body weight. Annu Rev Psychol 2000;51:255–77.
8. Lin J, Jiang Y, Wang G, et al. Associations of short sleep duration with appetite-regulating hormones and adipokines: a systematic review and meta-analysis. Obes Rev 2020;21(11):e13051.
9. Dahmen N, Bierbrauer J, Kasten M. Increased prevalence of obesity in narcoleptic patients and relatives. Eur Arch Psychiatry Clin Neurosci 2001; 251(2):85–9.
10. Schuld A, Hebebrand J, Geller F, et al. Increased body-mass index in patients with narcolepsy. Lancet 2000;355(9211):1274–5.
11. Sekine M, Yamagami T, Handa K, et al. A dose-response relationship between short sleeping hours and childhood obesity: results of the Toyama Birth Cohort Study. Child Care Health Dev 2002;28(2):163–70.
12. Deng X, He M, He D, et al. Sleep duration and obesity in children and adolescents: evidence from an updated and dose-response meta-analysis. Sleep Med 2021;78:169–81.
13. Simon SL, Diniz Behn C, Laikin A, et al. Sleep & circadian health are associated with mood & behavior in adolescents with overweight/obesity. Behav Sleep Med 2020;18(4):550–9.
14. Ludwig DS, Ebbeling CB. Type 2 diabetes mellitus in children: primary care and public health considerations. JAMA 2001;286(12):1427–30.
15. Daniels SR. The consequences of childhood overweight and obesity. Future Child 2006;16(1):47–67.
16. Mei H, Jiang F, Li L, et al. Study of genetic correlation between children's sleep and obesity. J Hum Genet 2020;65(11):949–59.
17. Bosy-Westphal A, Hinrichs S, Jauch-Chara K, et al. Influence of partial sleep deprivation on energy balance and insulin sensitivity in healthy women. Obes Facts 2008;1(5):266–73.
18. Nedeltcheva AV, Kilkus JM, Imperial J, et al. Sleep curtailment is accompanied by increased intake of calories from snacks. Am J Clin Nutr 2009;89(1): 126–33.
19. Locard E, Mamelle N, Billette A, et al. Risk factors of obesity in a five year old population. Parental versus environmental factors. Int J Obes Relat Metab Disord 1992;16(10):721–9.
20. Cappuccio FP, Taggart FM, Kandala NB, et al. Meta-analysis of short sleep duration and obesity in children and adults. Sleep 2008;31(5):619–26.
21. Bayon V, Leger D, Gomez-Merino D, et al. Sleep debt and obesity. Ann Med 2014;46(5):264–72.
22. Vgontzas AN, Fernandez-Mendoza J, Miksiewicz T, et al. Unveiling the longitudinal association between short sleep duration and the incidence of obesity: the Penn State Cohort. Int J Obes (Lond) 2014; 38(6):825–32.
23. Appelhans BM, Janssen I, Cursio JF, et al. Sleep duration and weight change in midlife women: the SWAN sleep study. Obesity (Silver Spring) 2013; 21(1):77–84.
24. Monti A, Doulazmi M, Nguyen-Michel VH, et al. Clinical characteristics of sleep apnea in middle-old and oldest-old inpatients: symptoms and comorbidities. Sleep Med 2021;82:179–85.
25. Simpson L, McArdle N, Eastwood PR, et al. Physical inactivity is associated with moderate-severe

obstructive sleep apnea. J Clin Sleep Med 2015; 11(10).1091–9.

26. West SD, Kohler M, Nicoll DJ, et al. The effect of continuous positive airway pressure treatment on physical activity in patients with obstructive sleep apnoea: a randomised controlled trial. Sleep Med 2009;10(9):1056–8.

27. Stevens D, Loffler KA, Buman MP, et al. CPAP increases physical activity in obstructive sleep apnea with cardiovascular disease. J Clin Sleep Med 2021; 17(2):141–8.

28. Drager LF, Brunoni AR, Jenner R, et al. Effects of CPAP on body weight in patients with obstructive sleep apnoea: a meta-analysis of randomised trials. Thorax 2015;70(3):258–64.

29. Redenius R, Murphy C, O'Neill E, et al. Does CPAP lead to change in BMI? J Clin Sleep Med 2008; 4(3):205–9.

30. Katz ES, Moore RH, Rosen CL, et al. Growth after adenotonsillectomy for obstructive sleep apnea: an RCT. Pediatrics 2014;134(2):282–9.

31. Crisafulli E, Beneventi C, Bortolotti V, et al. Energy expenditure at rest and during walking in patients with chronic respiratory failure: a prospective two-phase case-control study. PLoS One 2011;6(8): e23770.

32. Loring SH, Garcia-Jacques M, Malhotra A. Pulmonary characteristics in COPD and mechanisms of increased work of breathing. J Appl Physiol (1985) 2009;107(1):309–14.

33. Bonnet MH, Berry RB, Arand DL. Metabolism during normal, fragmented, and recovery sleep. J Appl Physiol (1985) 1991;71(3):1112–8.

34. Georgoulis M, Yiannakouris N, Kechribari I, et al. The effectiveness of a weight-loss Mediterranean diet/lifestyle intervention in the management of obstructive sleep apnea: results of the "MIMOSA" randomized clinical trial. Clin Nutr 2021;40(3):850–9.

35. Patel SR. The complex relationship between weight and sleep apnoea. Thorax 2015;70(3):205–6.

36. American Academy of Sleep Medicine. International Classification of sleep disorders. 3rd edition. Darien (IL): American Academy of Sleep Medicine; 2014.

37. Masa JF, Pépin JL, Borel JC, et al. Obesity hypoventilation syndrome. Eur Respir Rev 2019;28(151): 180097.

38. Wang Z, Wu H, Stone WS, et al. Body weight and basal metabolic rate in childhood narcolepsy: a longitudinal study. Sleep Med 2016;25:139–44.

39. Filardi M, Pizza F, Antelmi E, et al. Physical activity and sleep/wake behavior, anthropometric, and metabolic profile in pediatric narcolepsy type 1. Front Neurol 2018;9:707.

40. Sellayah D, Bharaj P, Sikder D. Orexin is required for brown adipose tissue development, differentiation, and function. Cell Metab 2011;14(4):478–90 [published correction appears in Cell Metab. 2012; 16(4):550].

41. Uchiyama M, Okawa M, Shibui K, et al. Poor recovery sleep after sleep deprivation in delayed sleep phase syndrome. Psychiatry Clin Neurosci 1999; 53(2):195–7.

42. Di Lorenzo L, De Pergola G, Zocchetti C, et al. Effect of shift work on body mass index: results of a study performed in 319 glucose-tolerant men working in a Southern Italian industry. Int J Obes Relat Metab Disord 2003;27(11):1353–8.

43. Sun M, Feng W, Wang F, et al. Meta-analysis on shift work and risks of specific obesity types. Obes Rev 2018;19(1):28–40.

44. Noh J. The effect of circadian and sleep disruptions on obesity risk. J Obes Metab Syndr 2018;27(2): 78–83.

45. Youngstedt SD, Goff EE, Reynolds AM, et al. Has adult sleep duration declined over the last 50+ years? Sleep Med Rev 2016;28:69–85.

46. Spiegel K, Leproult R, Van Cauter E. Impact of sleep debt on metabolic and endocrine function. Lancet 1999;354(9188):1435–9.

47. St-Onge MP, Grandner MA, Brown D, et al. Sleep duration and quality: impact on lifestyle behaviors and cardiometabolic health: a scientific statement from the American Heart association. Circulation 2016;134(18):e367–86.

9780323849814